SOCIOLOGY IN FOCUS SER
General Editor: Murray Moris

Sickness, Health and Medicine

Ursula Dobraszczyc

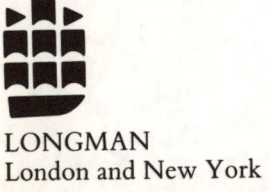

LONGMAN
London and New York

LONGMAN GROUP UK LIMITED
*Longman House, Burnt Mill, Harlow, Essex CM20 2JE, England
and Associated Companies throughout the World.*

**Published in the United States of America
by Longman Inc., New York.**

© **Longman Group UK Limited 1989**
*All rights reserved; no part of this publication
may be reproduced, stored in a retrieval system,
or transmitted in any form or by any means, electronic,
mechanical, photocopying, recording, or otherwise,
without the prior written permission of the Publishers,
or a licence permitting restricted copying issued by the
Copyright Licensing Agency Ltd, 90 Tottenham Court Road,
London, W1P 9HE.*

*First published 1989
Second impression 1992
ISBN 0 582 355354*

Set in 10/11pt Bembo, Linotron 202

Produced by Longman Singapore Publishers Pte Ltd

Printed in Singapore

British Library Cataloguing in Publication Data
Dobraszczyc, Ursula
 Sickness, health and medicine. – (Sociology in focus
series)
 1. Man. Health. Social aspects
 I. Title II. Series
 362.1'042

 ISBN 0–582–35535–4

*The publisher's policy is to use paper
manufactured from sustainable forests.*

Contents

Series introduction   v

Part 1   Introduction and overview

1   Introduction   1

Part 2   Sociological perspectives on medicine and health

2   Healing and scientific medicine   8
3   Health and industrialisation   22
4   Health inequalities   37
5   Being ill   57
6   Social control and medicine   72

Part 3   Statistical data and documentary readings

7   Statistical data   89
8   Documentary readings   102

Glossary of specialist terms   126
Bibliography   127
Index   128

For Julia Murphy and Jackie Groves

Series introduction

Sociology in Focus aims to provide an up-to-date, coherent coverage of the main topics that arise on an introductory course in sociology. While the intention is to do justice to the intricacy and complexity of current issues in sociology, the style of writing has deliberately been kept simple. This is to ensure that the student coming to these ideas for the first time need not become lost in what can appear initially as jargon.

Each book in the series is designed to show something of the purpose of sociology and the craft of the sociologist. Throughout the different topic areas the interplay of theory, methodology and social policy have been highlighted, so that rather than sociology appearing as an unwieldy collection of facts, the student will be able to grasp something of the process whereby sociological understanding is developed. The format of the books is broadly the same throughout. Part 1 provides an overview of the topic as a whole. In Part 2 the relevant research is set in the context of the theoretical, methodological and policy issues. The student is encouraged to make his or her own assessment of the various arguments, drawing on the statistical and reference material provided both here and at the end of the book. The final part of the book contains both statistical material and a number of 'Readings'. Questions have been provided in this section to direct students to analyse the materials presented in terms of both theoretical assumptions and methodological approaches. It is intended that this format should enable students to exercise their own sociological imaginations rather than to see sociology as a collection of universally accepted facts, which just have to be learned.

While each book in the series is complete within itself, the similarity of format ensures that the series as a whole provides an integrated and balanced introduction to sociology. It is intended that the text can be used both for individual and classroom study while the inclusion of the varied statistical and documentary materials lend themselves to both the preparation of essays and brief seminars.

PART 1
Introduction and overview

1   Introduction

To people living in pre-industrial Europe health meant soundness of mind and body or a state of physical and spiritual wellbeing sustained through God's grace. Since health was acknowledged to be a moral category there were few distinctions made between sinful and sickening activities, and disease was often understood to be a punishment. These ideas lasted well into modern times because, as K. Thomas says (*Religion and the Decline of Magic*, Penguin, 1978), the lives of the vast majority of the population were unaffected by the development of scientific medicine until well into the eighteenth century. Discoveries in medicine were of limited practical use, and financial and status considerations made the medical profession inaccessible to the mass of the people.

Traditional healing

In the past, as now, people used practical self-help to deal with problems of health. They had a repertoire of traditional remedies based on beliefs about the healing properties of plants and minerals which might be used in conjunction with special rituals, charms, prayers and spells. When these failed people consulted healers, and in doing so they drew no distinctions between the status of the cure offered by the physician, priest or herbalist. The latter, who were known as wise women and cunning men, used prayers to counteract the works of the Devil and his evil spirits, and practical remedies which could restore the balance of the body's humours. The prayer might be recited in Latin or written on a piece of paper to be burnt or hung round the neck of the afflicted animal or person.

Patient and healer alike believed that mythical events and holy names were a source of supernatural healing power. This can be illustrated by the special efficacy attributed to the 'Child's Prayer' which, when recited at the sick-bed, invoked the gospellers:

Matthew, Mark, Luke and John
Bless this bed that I lie on.

The Christian Church held that healing was part of the ministry and for this reason, and because of the belief that the forces of good and evil were involved in illness, it played a vital role in legitimising medical practices and practitioners.

Some people cured by touch alone. Until the end of the reign of Charles II, in 1689, it was believed that the monarch, as God's anointed, possessed healing powers, especially in relation to a kind of tuberculosis known as scrofula or 'The King's Evil'.

Cross-cultural comparison of healing

Anthropologists studying other cultures have documented systems of healing which are similar to those of pre-industrial Britain in that they combine elements regarded by contemporary medical practitioners as magical and religious with methods which are known to be 'effective'. E. E. Evans-Pritchard (*Witchcraft, Oracles and Magic among the Azande*, OUP, 1977, see Reading 1, p. 102) wrote that the Azande recognise two types of illness — one which can be treated by simple remedies because its origins are natural, and another which can be treated only by witchcraft and sorcery because it originates in the supernatural. The Azande perceive ritual and incantation as essential to the healing process and, furthermore, see no difference between what we might regard as 'effective methods' like washing a wound, and 'ineffective methods' such as placing a basket over the head of one's maternal uncle and pouring cold water over him to cure his nausea. (We could, however, pause to compare this method with the various remedies recommended for hiccups!)

Science and healing

Today, medical historians regard these forms of healing and the theories of illness which underpin them as pre-scientific: as belonging to societies which lack a knowledge of biology and disease mechanisms.

In industrialised societies we generally understand illness not to be the result of divine retribution or witchcraft. Our understanding of illness and health has been affected by the development of medical theories on the relationships between diet, life-style and environment under the impetus of the scientific revolution. The extent to which scientific rationality has actually displaced common-sense theories is a matter for debate, as we shall see in subsequent chapters. Still, it is possible to speak, as Kleinman does (A. Kleinman, *Patient and Healer in the Context of Culture*, University of California Press, 1980) of overlapping world-views in health care:

1 **the popular sector**, which is responsible, via such institutions as the family, for between 70 and 90 per cent of all health care through informal networks of people who share the same assumptions about staying healthy;
2 **the folk sector**, which rests upon holistic principles and is composed of people known as healers who may explicitly employ a mixture of the sacred and secular, faith and technical expertise to cure their clients; and
3 **the professional sector**, in which a collegiate body of professional healers practise within a legally defined monopoly.

The rise of professional medicine

From the seventeenth century to the nineteenth century, the medical profession in Britain gained a pre-eminence in matters of health. Its members won the right to be regarded as the experts — often at the expense of other practitioners such as herbalists, bonesetters and faith healers, and in the face of much popular opposition and mistrust. It was during this period that British society was transformed by the process of industrialisation, which initiated a series of changes bearing on the subject of health. Chief among them were changes in productivity and forms of work, the emergence of new classes and occupational groups (including the medical profession) and the creation of new forms of power, wealth and inequality. The benefits of the new industrial order were not evenly spread, and so health and income shared the same distribution curve as they do today. However, living standards generally rose, as did life expectancy.

Changes in the pattern of disease

The infectious diseases like typhus, cholera and tuberculosis ceased to be major causes of suffering and death. They have become known, along with the conditions directly produced by undernutrition, as the **diseases of poverty**. The main causes of death in industrial societies are cardio-vascular disease, cancer and the degenerative disorders collectively called the **diseases of affluence**. Most illnesses in contemporary Britain can be grouped into three types:

1 **chronic disease** – irreversible disorders such as bronchitis and arthritis which require supportive medical care;
2 **minor ailments** which are self-limiting, such as flu, chest infections and stress-related conditions which can be treated by drugs which are either self- or professionally prescribed;
3 **medico-surgical conditions** – curable if caught in time and constituting a tiny proportion of medical consultations and a high proportion of health expenditure. Where symptoms can be accepted and are acceptable in daily life they will be unreferred and unremarked; an example would be a 'smoker's cough'.

Illness today

Despite high living standards, the National Health Service and the medical profession, the population of Britain is not free of illness. The General Household Survey normally finds that up to 28 per cent of men and 30 per cent of women are suffering from a longstanding illness, 10 per cent of men and 14 per cent of women consult a doctor in the fourteen-day period prior to the interview and three-quarters receive a prescription. Many doctors regard these consultations as unnecessary since patients are presenting conditions that are either trivial or self-limiting. Yet sociologists have found in interviews outside of medical settings a **symptoms iceberg** of untreated illness in the ratio of one consultation to every ten cases of self-medication (K. Dunnell and A. Cartwright, *Medicine Takers, Prescribers and Hoarders*, RKP, 1972). D. R. Hannay in *The Symptoms Iceberg*, RKP, 1979, found from interviews with 1344 people, that 70 per cent of respondents who described themselves as being in 'good' or 'fair' health had symptoms for which there was serious pain and one in four had pain which was so severe that it caused inconvenience. It is not surprising that the best-selling proprietary drugs used in self-medication are the painkillers. Research by Dunnell and Cartwright (*Medicine Takers*) found that two out of three adults who said they were in 'excellent' health reported having had three or more clinical symptoms in the week preceding the interview, and 41 per cent of adults had taken some sort of analgesic, usually aspirin.

Conclusions

Two conclusions flow from the studies mentioned so far. First, the hope that advances in medical knowledge would produce a **healthy society** has not been realised. Second, **being healthy** is not our normal state and **being ill** the abnormal state brought about by bugs, viruses and bacteria. **Being sick** and **being well** are states affected by material, social and ideological factors, as the following points show.

First, in a study of general practice in South Wales, D. Robinson (*The Process of Becoming Ill*, RKP, 1971) found:

> Mrs M's account of her husband's leg injury illustrates the kind of manoeuvrings which were made around the notion of being ill and the role of the doctor.
>
> Mrs M: 'It wasn't too bad when he came in, just tender round the knee. It was stiff on Sunday and I said he'd have to go to the surgery on Monday . . . but he wouldn't. He started his new job with X's and you can't go sick on the first day . . . . Trust him to do it when he can't be on the sick. Next week he can make out he did it on the site. It's not that bad mind.' (He was

off work for two months as subsequent medical examination revealed serious ligament damage.

(D. Robinson, *The Process of Becoming Ill*, RKP, 1971, p. 14)

Second, most of the pharmacological preparations used in Britain are freely bought for self-medication from supermarkets and pharmacies by people who describe themselves as 'healthy'. People who have serious physical conditions may be unaware that they are ill until diagnosed as such by an expert. Healthy people who behave badly may be described as sick and subjected to **situation medicine**.

Third, although we are said to live in a scientific age, we do not approach sickness and health in a rational manner. We place great faith in the 'hot toddy', say 'Bless you' when somebody sneezes, and take medicines which make us feel better even though they are pharmacologically ineffective — and known to be so by the prescriber!

Fourth, many doctors feel that patients have become too dependent on the profession and fail to take responsibility for their own health. Many patients feel that their visit to the doctor has been successful only if it results in a prescription for medicines to be made up by the pharmacist. Yet, when 'conventional medicine' fails, sufferers still invoke the healing forces familiar to people in pre-industrial Britain (and Zande-land) by visiting faith healers, spiritualists and the sites of miraculous cures.

The organisation of this book

The relationship between health, illness, medicine and society are clearly complex, and the following chapters intend to show that sociological research does not support the widely held view that health is our normal state, illness is its opposite and the difference between the two is clear-cut even if it does require expert identification. Chapter 2 explores the factors giving rise to scientific medicine in the West and its relationship to other forms of healing. In Chapter 3 the relationships between health, illness and society are examined through a comparative study of health issues and the contribution of epidemiology. The main focus of Chapter 4 is inequalities in life chances as they have been described in recent studies of unemployment, poverty and access to structures of medical care. The social processes involved in referral and medical consultation are the concern of Chapter 5. Chapter 6 addresses the issue of medical power and the medicalisation of society through the study of mental illness and women's health. Chapters 7 and 8 present statistical and documentary material to complement and develop the themes which have been introduced in the preceding chapters.

PART 2
Sociological perspectives on medicine and health

2 Healing and scientific medicine

It is tempting, but unwise, to believe that because general improvements in health and declining mortality rates occurred at the same time as the emergence of scientific medicine, the former are the result of the latter. According to T. McKeown (*The Role of Medicine*, Basil Blackwell, 1979), the main factors determining physical health are nutrition, environment and individual behaviour — all of which the medical-care system and the individual practitioner were powerless to control because of their focus on the immediate symptoms of individual patients. Having examined mortality patterns since the nineteenth century he points out that, with the exception of diphtheria, medical science found ways of combating the most feared diseases only long after they had ceased to be major causes of death. The conditions successfully treated by medicine were those playing only a minor role in nineteenth-century mortality.

The observation that the reduction in mortality owes little to medical practice both challenges conventional wisdom and raises two sociologically important issues. The first of these is the influence of the medical profession's largely uncritical account of its history on our understanding of illness and health.

The second of the sociologically important issues is the relationship between illness and health and medicine both as a social institution and as a set of clinical practices.

Scientific progress

In presenting the history of medicine as a process of scientific

> Thomas Kuhn says that a science comes into being when disorganised sets of intellectual activities are united into an integrated body of techniques, assumptions and principles, which he calls **a paradigm**. The paradigm provides the framework within which research is undertaken. However, over time empirical evidence and theoretical problems will arise which it cannot contain. The cumulative exposure of deficiencies in the paradigm throws the scientific community out of the condition of normal science into a crisis phase. Revolutionary new principles are developed, and organised into a scheme which accommodates the new findings. A new paradigm replaces the old, and the scientific community re-writes the history of its discipline emphasising the continuities rather then the discontinuities between the new and the old, and the myth of smooth scientific progress is sustained.

discovery from quackery to science, medical historians have accomplished what Thomas Kuhn (*The Structure of Scientific Revolutions*, University of Chicago Press, 1970) says every scientific community sets out to do: they have emphasised the continuous and progressive nature of their discipline and excluded the embarrassing mistakes and blind alleys.

Pre-scientific medicine

In nineteenth-century medicine there were two important illustrations of Kuhn's ideas:

THE THEORY OF HUMOURS

This theory originated in ancient Greece and lingered well into the nineteenth century. It had provided a unified approach to the person in sickness and in health, linked the animate and inanimate worlds and incorporated astrology into healing practices. According to this approach, people were classified into four basic personality types depending on their normal balance of four elemental substances. Illness followed any disturbance of this balance, and the task of the diagnostician was to identify the disequilibrium and administer the appropriate remedy, often in the form of 'cooling' or 'heating' or 'purging' foods.

> The theory of humours yielded the following scheme:
> fire = yellow bile: hot and dry; choleric personality (spleen)
> earth = black bile: cold and dry; melancholy personality (liver)
> air = blood: hot and moist; sanguine personality (heart)
> water = phlegm: cold and moist; phlegmatic personality (brain)

The influence of humoural ideas can be seen in nineteenth-century treatments for cholera. As it was believed that uncontrollable excretion of fluids indicated an excess of moisture, the orthodox remedy was bleeding and purging with emetics. These traditional practices exacerbated the potentially fatal process of dehydration initiated by the illness and survived even in the face of contradictory evidence. A practitioner working during the 1831–32 outbreak had noticed that the blood of the afflicted was thicker and of a different composition than normal blood, and he reasoned that transfusions of fluids and salts would combat the disease. This remedy was theoretically sound even though its effectiveness was limited by practical deficiencies: poor equipment, inadequate sterilisation leading to a high risk of infection, the trial and error element in mixing up the correct salt and water solution and the fact that as a treatment of last resort it may have been administered to people too ill to recover. The treatment was publicised in *The Lancet* (quoted in R. J. Morris, *Cholera 1832*, Croom Helm, 1976) and then forgotten. Nearly a century later in Calcutta, between 1906 and 1920, the technique was developed, and mortality was reduced from 59 to 14 per cent.

CONTAGION AND MIASMA
Until the middle of the last century there were two competing theories of epidemic disease: **contagion**, the transmission of illness between people and animals by some unknown mechanism associated with physical contact (see Reading 2, p. 103; and **miasma**,

foul air emanating from rotting matter because of a natural disaster or the carnage of war elsewhere on earth.

The work of Louis Pasteur and Paul Koch on bacteria or 'microbes' (the 'little animals' that had puzzled scientists from the 1830s onwards) established **the doctrine of specific etiology**: that is, the theory that each specific illness has a specific cause. This firmly put an end to miasma theory and ushered in the modern 'germ theory of disease' which was to reign supreme for thirty years between 1870 and 1900, by which time changing patterns of illness implicated other factors. Today 'miasma' is regarded as a blind alley and lives on only in advertisements for air fresheners.

The development of scientific approaches

Pursuing the distinction made at the start of this chapter between therapeutic practices and the institution of medicine, how did the present structures come into being? Modern medicine divides healing practices into three types:

1 orthodox — scientific,
2 unorthodox — unscientific, and
3 quackery — mumbo-jumbo.

The categories owe less to therapeutic superiority than to the social status of practitioner and client. As Mary Chamberlain says in *Old Wives' Tales*:

> Medicine, like war, is an extension of politics. The story of the Old Wife isn't the story of an inferior practice losing ground with the advancement of medical science and technology, rather it is a story which concerns the politics of medicine — a story of control and access.
> (M. Chamberlain, *Old Wives' Tales*, Virago, 1981, p. 139)
> (See Reading 3, p. 104.)

Towards the end of the eighteenth century some of the diagnostic techniques still used by doctors were becoming known, such as auscultation (listening to the sounds of respiration and heartbeat) and percussion (tapping the chest in order to locate areas of congestion). But although the stethoscope had been introduced (in 1816 by René Laënnec) along with the thermometer, the pulse watch and mechanisms for measuring blood pressure, they were not widely used by physicians, who held aloof from machines and manual techniques which might associate them with tradesmen.

By 1800, lacking effective diagnostic aids and an understanding of illness as a physical state, physicians were limited to the alleviation of symptoms. Furthermore, the pharmacologies used by licensed practitioners were often exactly the same as those used in folk-medicine by wise women and quacks: opium, cascara, digitalis, 'crabs' eyes' and 'rose elixir'.

A scientific professional community can hardly be said to have existed at this stage, even though the Royal College of Physicians had occupied a prominent social position since the seventeenth century. Many of the discoveries which advanced medical care were not made by practitioners but by chemists and physicists working in laboratories, and both technical and institutional limitations hindered the flow of ideas between scientific workers. As R. H. Shryock says (*The Development of Modern Medicine*, University of Wisconsin, 1979), by the eighteenth century 'Physick lagged behind Physics'. But by the end of the nineteenth century medicine had technical, scientific and ideological support for its claims to expertise.

Shryock believes that scientific medicine came into being when physicians abandoned 'heroic medicine' (see Reading 4, p. 105) as exemplified by the practices of the American Benjamin Rush — the harsh therapeutics of bleeding, purging and the use of mineral preparations (mainly mercury). Although the new approaches entailed no major advances in treatment, they rested on a scientific perspective on the body as a mechanism.

Developments in anatomical knowledge

By 1800 medical men's claim to scientific status lay in their knowledge of 'gross anatomy' — that which could be seen with the naked eye — and from the year of the Anatomy Act, 1832, which legalised the dissection of the human body, they began to forge connections between the symptoms of sickness in the living and the state of their tissues in death.

From the 1840s onwards microbiology entered the field of medical knowledge because of improvements in lens-grinding techniques and advances in optical knowledge which, for example, reduced distortion and allowed people to study structures smaller than amoebae. Research into the structure and function of tissues and organs was further advanced by the staining of specimens with the aniline dyes which had been developed for the textile industry. In 1858, when Rudolph Virchow published *Cellular Pathology*, cell abnormality became the key to understanding disease, because he showed that disease processes can be observed through the microscope as cell changes.

New therapeutics

Separately, between 1857 and 1876 Louis Pasteur in France and Robert Koch in Germany studied micro-organisms and established their role in putrefaction and in the transmission of disease. Koch proved a causal relationship between illness and micro-organisms by injecting a healthy animal with a culture of anthrax, then drawing off blood samples from the afflicted beast to show the presence of the same micro-organism. From research of this kind, chemical therapeutics were linked to physical studies.

The tendency today is to see an activity as scientific to the degree that it uses quantification. However, as the examples quoted above show, the development of medical science depended more on experimental technique, controlled trials and the study of anatomy than quantification. In a sense medicine was a pure science in as far as the accumulation of scientific knowledge had no immediate impact on the lives of the mass of the people.

Ironically, there was one branch of medicine which depended upon quantitative techniques and which, according to McKeown (*The Role of Medicine*) made a clear contribution to the health of people in nineteenth-century Britain. This was the low status specialism of **epidemiology** or 'medical geography', as it was called. The impact of epidemiology is discussed in the next chapter in relation to the public health movement, but for the moment it is important to note that the study of tissues and the disease mechanism laid the foundation for modern medical science, and the introduction of antisepsis and anaesthesia ushered in the modern age of curative medical practice.

The branch of medicine which benefited most from these developments was surgery – the descendant of a very lowly specialism. Surgery had historically been a treatment of last resort and dealt mainly with the amputation of limbs which had become diseased or injured in accidents or wars. Its practitioners preferred to rely upon speed and the traditional intoxicants of opium and alcohol, even though, according to Shryock (*The Development of Modern Medicine*) the sleep-inducing properties of nitrous oxide had been known since the early 1800s. Unfortunately for another group of practitioners who, unlike the surgeons, hoped to see their patients more than once, the effects of alcohol and opium were limited and unpredictable. It was the teeth-pullers or dentists, as they were to be known, who promoted anaesthesia with nitrous oxide, ether and, later, chloroform. The great advantage of the anaesthetic, apart from patient comfort and reduced operative shock, was that it gave the surgeon time. From the 1840s onwards surgery became more commonplace but so did death from infection, as post-operative deaths from 'hospital fever' ran at 10 per cent.

Some of the medical advances provoked moral debate. In obstetric medicine pain relief was a controversial issue since the Biblical text, 'in sorrow shalt thou bring forth children', had created a class of patients for whom pain was prescribed — pregnant women! Theories of motherhood even held that a woman would not feel real affection for her child if she had a painless delivery. In 1853, at the birth of her eighth child, Queen Victoria gave obstetric anaesthesia the Royal seal of approval.

The growth of the medical profession

Alongside these developments in scientific knowledge, changes were occurring in the three closed status groups which laid claim to medical orthodoxy: the Royal College of Physicians, the Royal College of Surgeons, and the Worshipful Company of Apothecaries. They came into conflict with one another for status, clients, legitimacy and autonomy at the same time as opposing and devaluing practitioners outside of their organisations. Modern medicine emerged as a social institution largely through the strategies adopted by these three groups in relation to one another and to the powerful interests of the day.

The physicians, surgeons and apothecaries were functionally differentiated and had protected legal status. With their own governing bodies, foremost of which was the Royal College of Physicians, they set tests of competence and they controlled training and conduct. By the middle of the eighteenth century when the idea of the professional gentleman arose, its members served the upper classes. This was a small group whose values and manners physicians shared. The intimacy of relationships with patients often meant that social acceptability counted for more than technical competence. The characteristics of a good physician were a university education and a good bedside manner. This stage of professional development is called **bedside medicine** by N. Jewson ('Medical Knowledge and the Patronage System in Eighteenth-century England', *Sociology*, vol. 8, no. 3, Sept. 1974). Symptoms and treatments had to be negotiated with the patient, who held the balance of power in the relationship partly by virtue of economic superiority and partly because of the limited effectiveness of medical practice at this time.

Physicians tried to maintain a strict division of labour between themselves and the surgeons and apothecaries. The former were men of limited education who worked with their hands often as 'field doctors' for the military and belonged to the Guild which included barbers and teeth-pullers. Their claim to professional status was advanced by the establishment of medical schools whose curriculum included the study of practical anatomy and pathology.

Apothecaries had belonged to the Grocers' Guild, and their association with trade as dispensers of drugs, nostrums and quack remedies made them the social inferiors of physicians. But from the middle of the seventeenth century they had engaged in diagnosis and treatment mainly on behalf of the growing middle-class population which was socially and financially excluded from the physician's practice.

The divisions among these groups began to break down as a result of population growth that, along with economic growth, increased the size of the provincial middle class which demanded medical care of a general kind. The metropolitan bodies could no longer regulate the regions, and provincial associations were springing up all over Britain. This was most marked in the case of the apothecaries, who were the closest equivalent to today's general practitioner and whose numbers exceeded those of physicians in 1794. The table on page 16, quoted in an article in the *Westminster Review*, vol. 45, 1846, p. 57, gives figures for 1841.

During the first thirty years of the century the Guild was no longer seen to be an appropriate model for medical occupations and various proposals to reorganise medicine were put forward —

The medical profession, 1841

	England	Wales	Scotland	Ireland	British Isles	United Kingdom
Physicians	1,063	30	364	300	19	1,776
Surgeons and apothecaries	14,102	526	2,237	2,100	141	19,106
Medical students	1,320	76	248	500	8	2,152
Total	16,485	632	2,849	2,900	168	23,034

usually with physicians in command. The Medical Registration Act of 1858 created a unified medical profession which incorporated the physicians, apothecaries and surgeons and established the General Council of Medical Education and Regulation, which had four main purposes. These were

1 to maintain a register of licensed practitioners;
2 to determine the level and nature of qualifications appropriate for registration;
3 to obtain where necessary the co-operation of the examining bodies; and
4 to appoint examiners.

The next stage in the development of the medical profession occurred when the locus of medical work shifted from the home to the hospital. This transformation was important both clinically and socially: medicine acquired an institutional identity, and doctors became increasingly involved with new classes of patient who were usually their social inferiors.

Although, as in the past, the majority of people had little contact with the profession since it was not part of a public service in the accepted sense, there was a variety of medical institutions for those who did receive medical treatment: old-established **voluntary hospitals** maintained by public subscription and taking patients who had acceptable references; **teaching hospitals** which catered for cases with an educational value and specialist institutions, such as **fever hospitals**, **lying-in hospitals**, and **free dispensaries** for the poor and wards administered by the District Medical Officer appointed under the Poor Laws.

The voluntary hospitals were important to the profession because, where they were linked to medical schools, they offered a corporate identity in addition to training opportunities. During their training, medical students learned to regard diagnosis as an objective activity and medical practice as oriented to the case rather than the individual. Further, the invitation to practise in a voluntary hospital brought the newly qualified physician into contact with wealthy patrons who were potential clients.

The final stage is **laboratory medicine**. Although most medical work does not actually involve high technology and 'wonder drugs and cures', it is nevertheless located within an ideological context of scientific advance. The modern medical practitioner is under considerably more pressure to make people well than in the past, when fatalism prevailed. Some commentators have detected a consumerist trend in public attitudes which may threaten the security of the medical profession. However, history provides ample evidence for the claim that the status and authority of the medical profession have never been entirely secure.

A challenge to professional authority

In his study of class relations during the 1831–32 cholera outbreak, R. J. Morris (*Cholera 1832*) explored the factors affecting official and popular responses to the epidemic and the social position of doctors. As they charted the progress of Asiatic cholera across Europe towards Britain, the authorities devised some protective measures but no firm policies. Fearing the worst, and mindful that the Black Death of 1349 nearly halved Europe's population, the government set up an Inspectorate with Local and National Boards of Health to monitor the epidemic and make appropriate arrangements.

The two theories of epidemic diseases mentioned above had different policy implications. **Miasma** led to public cleansing and the care of the sick. **Contagion** led to isolation of the sick and the quarantine of affected areas. Professional divisions in support for these theories produced a variety of responses. In some areas support for contagion resulted in conflict with local mercantile interests. In seaports, for example, where physicians had a place in the business community by virtue of status or because they were part-owners in ships or cargoes, there was a lot at risk if quarantine were used to halt the spread of cholera.

When the first suspected case appeared in Sunderland the authorities were reluctant to make a firm diagnosis. Symptoms could be confused with those of 'summer fever' or the familiar condition going by the name of 'English cholera'. The only people with experience of cholera and competent in diagnosis were often the army doctors whose low status gave them little credibility with local physicians.

Official action was regarded with suspicion by the public since the outbreak coincided with two controversial pieces of legislation: the Anatomy Act and the Great Reform Bill. Radicals were inclined to view government warnings and public health measures as plots by the ruling class against the reform movement. Activists countered what they saw as propaganda by encouraging people to come to rallies and public meetings but to use vinegar sprays as protection against infection. As the epidemic became established, other reformers made much of the very obvious class-gradient in suffering and death. And in addition, the leaders of the nascent Temperance movement pronounced the disease to be God's punishment for the intemperate.

Today we know that, because cholera is actually a difficult disease for healthy people to catch, it is a good indicator of ill health and malnutrition. However, during the 1832 outbreak, 32 000 people were estimated to have died and many more were exposed to the vibrio but were healthy enough to survive. Doctors were unable to halt or cure the illness, and the public health measures they introduced were often unpopular. For example, the regulations meant that the corpse of a cholera victim had to be removed for official burial within twenty-four hours. According to Morris, this struck against the burial practices of the poor. They needed time to arrange funerals, which were usually held on everyone's day off – Sunday. People needed to sort out finances and arrange for friends and relatives to pay their last respects.

Conflict was exacerbated by a provision of the Anatomy Act allowing doctors to claim for scientific research the bodies of people who had died in hospital or the workhouse if neither they nor their relatives had indicated any objection. There were public demonstrations against doctors, who became the target of working-class hostility, and people feared for themselves and their relatives if they were taken into quarantine as suspected cases. Tales of 'corpses' being taken by cart for dissection in laboratories suddenly showing signs of life entered the folklore of medical horror stories. Popular distrust of the medical profession, despite its role in the undoubtedly beneficial public health movement, was fuelled by specific events such as those described and, more generally, by the contradiction between the ideology of public service and the reality of a free market in health care which resulted in automatic treatment for those who could afford it and uncertainty for everyone else.

Sociology of the profession

The division discussed above between how the profession presented itself and how it was regarded by many outsiders is mirrored by the two traditions in the sociology of the professions.

Trait theory

Professions are seen as occupational groups characterised by a set of distinctive features. They possess a specialist body of knowledge imparted to students over a long period of training. Practitioners are bound by a code of ethics which entails (in the interest of patients) the protection of clinical freedom from outside interference, the maintenance of confidentiality and a respect for the trust placed in doctors because patients lack the knowledge by which to judge medical competence. The profession has its own regulatory body which sets standards and has the power to discipline or expel errant members. High salaries and status are the rewards earned by the skill and integrity of the professional.

Professionalism as a market strategy

Professionalism is a market strategy which promotes and secures the interests of an occupational group. By controlling entry, the group controls labour supply and ensures that there is never a surplus to threaten the livelihoods of those currently practising. Doctors control the activities of members in the interests of the profession as a whole but claim that public and professional interests coincide. Conduct which is morally reprehensible is punished, but technical incompetence escapes notice because of clinical freedom and the unwillingness of one doctor to interfere in another's case. The sole right to practise granted by the 1858 Medical Registration Act, for example, gave doctors the power to determine the shape of the National Health Service in 1948 and their own position of privilege within it.

Lay and scientific healing

This last approach is taken by Chamberlain (*Old Wives' Tales*) in her account of how the medical profession (1) denied women access to the forms of training upon which scientific medicine was based, and (2) devalued the traditional remedies used by women at the same time as they were being incorporated into orthodox therapies. She says that healing was an extension of women's domestic role and, to the working class especially, women's folk-remedies were effective, cheap and accessible. Professional men reacted to this emerging clash of interests by policies of exclusion and denial. Women were excluded from more than an occupation; they were excluded from the scientific community whose theories and paradigms came to provide ideological justification for the social inferiority of women.

Another social group which benefited from the disappearance of the wise women was pharmacy: retail chemists. Their small businesses, selling preparations made up behind the counter, provided medical aid for working-class people to whom illness meant destitution and the workhouse. Although the stories of Beecham's (Little Liver Pills — worth a guinea a box) and Boot's are another chapter in the development of medicine, quackery and the commercialisation of folk healing, the reader might like to consider at this point the relationships between medical practice, pharmacy and the food and drug industries.

The case of homoeopathy

Other groups, known as **the irregulars**, had their fortunes changed by the professionalisation of medicine in the nineteenth century. They included osteopaths and homoeopaths.

In his history of homoeopathy, H. L. Coulter in *The Divided*

Legacy (North Atlantic Books, 1982) says that the debate between homoeopathy and what became known as orthodox medicine involves the meaning of science itself, because homoeopathy involves a unique theory of cause and effect in illness as well as its own paradigm of health and healing.

Samuel Hahnemann, a doctor and pharmacologist born in 1755, is acknowledged to be the founder of this form of healing which is based on the principle of **similars** rather than **contraries** or **allopathy**.

The homoeopath pursues a holistic approach, looking beyond the immediate symptoms to the dynamic pattern of symptoms in relation to the person as an individual. The healer tries to discover why the body's life-force is disturbed, and then administers preparations to stimulate natural defences. In a state of health people coexist with all kinds of germs and bacteria without being affected, so ill health has more to do with the person than with infection by germs. Hahnemann condemned heroic medicine as nonsense, and argued that effective treatments depend on a secure knowledge of the body's own healing mechanisms.

The homoeopathic theory of ill health leads to gentle therapeutics — preparations are based on natural substances which have been 'proved' on healthy people, they are not addictive, they do not have side effects and it is impossible to overdose. But because therapy is patient-, rather than symptom-centred it is not susceptible to the types of random-controlled trials by which the efficacy of treatment is scientifically established. Homoeopathy went into relative decline when the work of people such as Pasteur and Koch lent powerful support to the germ theory of illness.

So, by the end of the century the structure of the medical profession and its authority in all matters of physical and mental well-being were established.

3 Health and industrialisation

This chapter explores the relationships between illness, health and economic change by looking at Britain and comparing its past and present with poor countries today. These issues will be addressed after a consideration of **epidemiology**, which has always informed debates in this area through the collection of statistical data on life chances, mortality and access to resources such as money and food.

Epidemiology

When John Snow removed the handle from the Broad Street water pump in the Soho district of London during the 1853–54 cholera outbreak, he had no proof that cholera was a water-borne disease. But he had analysed the city's cholera maps of 1849 charting the incidence of notified cases, and he argued that there was a pattern in the distribution of cholera suggestive of a relationship between the disease and domestic water supplies. The Broad Street outbreak was confined to about 500 people living in an area 250 yards across who were all clients of one of the two water companies supplying the area. The one victim who lived outside of the neighbourhood was a woman who liked the taste of the water from the Broad Street pump so much that she had it transported to her home. Snow's action meant that the pump could not be used and so, as the source of infection was closed off, the incidence of cholera declined. Later investigation revealed that the drinking water had been contaminated by sewage through a broken conduit.

Snow's work is regarded as a classic in epidemiology: the tradition of 'medical mapping' or 'medical geography' which began at the turn of the eighteenth century. During the nineteenth century, data on health and illness were compiled by three main groups:

1 medical practitioners using their case notes to explore disease mechanisms;

2 campaigners such as Edwin Chadwick, using data on disease to prove that governments could raise standards of individual health by introducing public health measures; and
3 academics studying the relationships between disease, population growth and economic development.

By today's standards the data and statistical techniques available to researchers in the nineteenth century leave a lot to be desired. There were no sources of reliable figures produced in continuous series enabling comparison to be made over time. However, the collection of 'vital statistics' (information on birth, marriage, death and disease) was increasingly regarded as an aspect of government, an adjunct to medical science and a justification for social science.

Today, epidemiologists use data which are either produced by large-scale medical surveys or collected by official bodies such as governments and the World Bank. They make correlations between variables in order to suggest or establish causes of social and medical problems. Epidemiology is of interest to sociologists for two perhaps contradictory reasons; both are illustrated by the contents of this chapter. On the one hand, in the positivist traditions of the last century, sociologists accept epidemiological data as valid and use them in the study of social problems – class patterns in illness, for example. On the other hand, sociologists make epidemiological data the object of their study in exploring the role of statistical information in the social construction of reality. The two main assumptions upon which epidemiology rests – that official statistics can be regarded as a record of human action, and that aspects of human action can be meaningfully recorded and counted by official bodies – raise questions about causal relationships and the social processes involved in structuring data which are themselves of interest to sociology.

There are always questions about the validity of epidemiological data, whether they relate to 'soft' statistics such as delinquency or comparatively 'hard' data such as death rates. Delinquency is a social category involving socially structured forms of evaluation and classification because figures are determined by the conceptual frameworks of the collecting agencies. All deaths have to be registered, and so the relationship between mortality and its record is closer than is the case between delinquent behaviour and the statistics. Death certificates record the occurrence and place of a death as well as its primary and associated causes. Nevertheless, data on the nature and cause of death are influenced by the same kinds of processes as those operating in the case of delinquency. Doctors faced with the same symptoms, history and signs will often reach different conclusions. If the errors are random, then they probably would not cause concern except where highly dangerous or work-related conditions were a possibility. But are there patterns in the errors?

Cameron and McGoogan in a study of 1 152 hospital deaths in Scotland (*Journal of Pathology*, 1981, vol. 133, pp. 273−83) compared autopsy and death certificates, and found clinical diagnosis to be correct in 61 per cent cases but wrong in 39 per cent of cases. Accuracy was high in thoracic cases but low in infections and cerebro-vascular illness. Accuracy had an inverse relationship with age and length of stay in hospital: high in patients under forty-five years (78 per cent cases), low in patients over seventy-five years (less than 50 per cent). They found two types of discrepancy:

1 **overdiagnosis**, where the clinical cause of death was not confirmed at autopsy (in 27 per cent of the main cause of death) and where the condition was present but was not confirmed by the pathologist as the cause of death; and
2 **underdiagnosis**, where a diagnosis made at autopsy had not been clinically anticipated − this was most frequent in infections (62 per cent of cases) and cardio-vascular illness (67 per cent of cases).

Among other reasons, the discrepancies are notable because in 58 per cent of cases it is suggested that different procedures should have been followed; 52 per cent should have had different treatment and in 61 per cent of cases unnecessary or dangerous treatment was given. Those dying within three days had high rates of confirmation perhaps because there was a clear cause for admission in the first place (66 per cent). Long hospital stays were associated with a fall in requests for autopsy, and yet this area had the greatest degree of discrepancy. In 56 per cent of these cases the discrepancy involved a change in the main cause of death. It could be argued that long-stay hospital patients are likely also to be elderly people whose multiple pathologies make diagnosis difficult, but the marked discrepancies began at fifty-four years of age. One tentative suggestion is that we may be systematically underestimating infection in our morbidity and mortality statistics because of its association with underdevelopment.

The advantages of the epidemiological approach

The epidemiological approach is valuable because it can be an alternative to laboratory work. Studies on the large scale may generate hypotheses and multi-factorial theories which would not emerge from small-scale case studies. Long-term studies can be undertaken relatively inexpensively and without raising the ethical questions which are involved in experiments on animals and people. There are three other advantages for medical research: first, the study of people in natural settings; second, the focus on, or selection of, particular attributes which may deserve further study; and third, the provision of forms of quantitative data not available in laboratory studies and detail on very small effects.

The disadvantages of epidemiological approaches

There are theoretical, empirical and ethical disadvantages. How does one distinguish between a causal relationship and a spurious connection? Has one taken into consideration confounding factors which may have occurred in both data collection and analysis? Finally, data relevant to epidemiological investigation will always be collected according to current theories.

Illustration of all of these points can be given from the report of the *British Empire Cancer Campaign* produced in 1937. The author, who was one of the pioneers of demography, explained that his maps showing the age and sex distribution of cancer excluded people under twenty-five years of age because the 'risk of dying of cancer of most organs is very small at ages under 25 years but rises very rapidly with advancing age to a maximum at about 70 years or later' (P. Stocks, vol. 14, p. 259). He went on to say that 'Cancer deaths before 25 years of age comprise only an insignificant fraction of all cancer deaths, moreover, some 3/4 of them are from sarcoma contrasted with only 40% at ages after 25 years so the causative factors are probably somewhat different from those usually concerned in producing cancer at a more advanced age' (p. 260).

Today cancer is the second most important cause of death in the age group 5–25 years. Have the young experienced a sharper increase in cancers than the older populations in the last fifty years, or was there a failure to diagnose the cancers of the young in the

1930s because of the then prevalent view that cancer was a disease of the old? (see Reading 5, p. 106.)

Epidemiology can never entirely substitute for laboratory studies because it is important to show that the correlation for the group also holds true for the individual case. Observations are always limited to events that have already occurred along a time scale, which means that by the time research is published there may have been considerable anguish and suffering. Nevertheless, McKeown places epidemiology at the centre of the movement for public health and disease prevention. It was one of the elements in the process by which private affairs became seen as both a matter of public concern and state regulation.

Living standards and health in Britain

The nineteenth century

Epidemiological work demonstrated that the same factors as those identified by the World Health Organisation in the struggle for 'Health for all for the year 2000' – **sanitation, pure water** and **nutrition** were the main determinants of life-chances in nineteenth-century England. The development of the British economy was associated with a fall in death rate from 32 per 1 000 in 1750 to 23 per 1 000 a century later and 18 per 1 000 in 1900.

> Birth, death and migration affect the size and composition of the population. Changes in size and composition affect in turn social needs and institutional structures. Compare, for example, the health-care needs of societies with large proportions of young people or older people.
>
> Statistics on births are generally presented as two rates:
>
> 1 The crude birth rate (CBR) is the number of live births in a year per 1 000 people in the population. For example, from 1850 to 1930 Britain's CBR dropped from 35/1 000 to 15/1 000 mainly because people adopted contraceptive

> techniques to determine when, and how many, children they would have. As CBR is based on total population (women, children and men), it can give a distorted picture of reproductive behaviour.
> 2 A better picture can be drawn from the rates of birth in relation to maternal age — the age-specific birth rate.
>
> Fertility is a major factor affecting the size of population, whereas composition is heavily influenced by mortality. Four sets of mortality figures are of particular interest in the study of health: crude death rate, infant mortality rate (the number of children dying in the first year of life relative to the number of births), age-specific mortality and standardised mortality ratios. The latter allows for peculiarities in the age structure of a local population to be taken into account when large-scale comparisons are to be made. It involves a relative standard — 100 represents the average, and figures for localities are calculated in relation to it: 125 is above average and 75 below.
>
> After 1850 the mortality data for all classes in Britain improved. The crude death rate fell by a third between 1889 to 1911 to hover around 11/1 000. The most substantial drop occurred in infant mortality, which is generally considered to be the most sensitive index of health in a society. So, although fewer children were born per woman, more survived into adulthood and old age. At the turn of the century Britain had a young population — one-third of the population was under fifteen years, whereas today a quarter are over sixty. However, two points need to be remembered. First, the death rates did not decline in a uniform manner, which shows that the factors involved in the health and death of men, women and children are not the same; and second, the class-gradient in population and health statistics did not disappear, which shows that 'life-chances' are not evenly distributed.

This fall is attributed mainly to a decline in infectious diseases: even before the development of effective medical treatment death from TB was declining, and this reduction accounted for 50 per cent of the drop in the death rate. Reductions in deaths from typhus and scarlet fever account for 20 per cent, from cholera, dysentery and diarrhoea for 10 per cent and from smallpox for 5 per cent. Refinements in diagnosis and classification may have altered the figures because, for example, leprosy, syphilis and smallpox were often confused, but in general as nutritional standards rose and forms of environmental control were introduced the health of the population improved. The general principle is that people who are adequately fed have a higher resistance to infections and parasites than those who are not.

The illnesses currently called **the diseases of underdevelopment** were once either endemic or epidemic in Britain: cholera, typhoid and typhus, malaria, plague, hookworm, tapeworm, tetanus, smallpox and leprosy. They are not tropical diseases in the sense of being somehow produced by, and confined to, areas with a tropical climate; they are the diseases of poverty.

The wealthy classes in nineteenth-century Britain equated industrial capitalism with progress, and were either ignorant of its human costs or preferred to regard them as unavoidable and as aggravated by working-class fecklessness. However, some people, acting out of philanthropy or self-interest, fought for reforms which reduced morbidity and mortality.

A major figure in this connection was Edwin Chadwick, the main author of the 1842 Report on the Sanitary Conditions of the Labouring Population of Great Britain and the advocate of a national system of water supply and sewage disposal. Gradually, permissive legislation (for example, the Vaccination Act of 1840 empowering parish guardians to provide free smallpox vaccination on request) was replaced by legal requirement (compulsory smallpox vaccination for infants less than three months old, under the 1853 Vaccination Act), and a national system of regulatory bodies responsible for public health was set up.

These measures did not meet with unequivocal popular support. Engels wrote in 1845 that the urban poor viewed the authorities as agents of control and repression rather than improvement. Indeed, the correct terms for public health officials at this time were 'the sanitary police' and 'the medical police'.

Occasionally when an epidemic threatens, the otherwise sleepy conscience of the sanitary police is a little stirred, raids are made into the working-men's districts, whole rows of cellars and cottages are closed; but this does not last long: the condemned

cottages soon find occupants again, the owners are much better off by letting them, and the sanitary police won't come again so soon.
(F. Engels, *The Condition of the Working-class in England in 1844*, Lawrence & Wishart, 1954, p. 93)

Engels' work represents an alternative to the reformist tradition of the day because he locates the source of squalor and ill health in the dynamics of capitalism rather than in the culture of the poor.

Turning to the role of nutrition, it is important to go beyond the generalisation that 'nutritional standards rose', but it is a difficult task because of confusing and contradictory claims. Obtaining and interpreting the information is not easy. Clearly, the quantity and variety of foods available were increased with improvements in trade and production so that the prospect of famine receded. However, evidence on the gap between the resources of the rich and the poor suggest that malnutrition did not disappear (see Reading 6, p. 107). In some respects people's diets a hundred years ago were more healthy than they are today because of the high consumption of unrefined foods, and yet food was less pure than it is today because it was not produced to the standards of hygiene we are accustomed to.

Today life-style and diet play an important part in our theories of disease. This may be due to the fact that infections which were the scourge of the nineteenth century are much more amenable to contemporary medical care than are the degenerative disorders which account for so much contemporary illness. Because heart disease and cancer have complex causalities and uncertain treatments diet has come to be seen as playing a part in prevention if not also in cause and cure.

Industrialisation brought changes to the production and consumption of food. Quantity and variety, though not always quality, were increased by the commercialisation of agriculture and the exploitation of colonial territories. At the end of the eighteenth century many Britons had still produced much of their own food through small-scale vegetable and animal husbandry. Indeed, notwithstanding the sanitary regulations, the practice of rearing pigs, chickens and rabbits in back yards was carried on by workers in some manufacturing towns late into the nineteenth and early twentieth centuries. During the nineteenth century, as Burnett shows (*Plenty and Want*, Scholar Press, 1979), increases in population and incomes stimulated demand. Patterns of work and domestic life changed and, consequently, so did eating habits and nutritional standards. As food processing and retailing became big businesses, the incentives and structural pre-conditions for food adulteration came into being. Competition, the ideology of *laissez-faire*, taxes on many staple foods, small profit margins and long chains of control from producer to consumer meant that widespread, undetectable and profitable adulteration took place. Some additives were simply cheaper, inferior substitutes making the product go further. Some were poisonous or affected the body in a cumulative way as with copper and arsenic commonly used to colour sweets and tea. Food manufacturers devised new methods of food preservation and enhancement using chemicals, canning and refrigeration.

The Chartist demand for cheap, good food was kept alive as a political issue by the Co-operative movement. But there was some reluctance to buy 'pure' food; people were used to the taste, colour and cost of the adulterated varieties. They had to be persuaded that tea tasted better if it was not artificially tinted bright green and that bread baked from flours artificially whitened was harmful. The Co-op Central Agency, formed in 1850, even employed lecturers to 'educate working-class palates'.

Then, as now, poverty produced large pockets of undernourishment. An interdepartmental committee on physical deterioration was set up in 1904, and found that one in three children were suffering from malnutrition. Their inquiries were initiated after 50 per cent of recruits for the Boer War were found to be in poor health or of unsatisfactory physique. The malnutrition of the poor was accentuated by food-poverty between members of poor families, as the Women's Co-operative Guild showed. Women stretched their housekeeping by giving priority to their husbands and children and by going without themselves. Maternal malnutrition and overwork were identified as the chief causes of infant and maternal mortality and ill health. The Women's Co-operative Guild campaigned for food, money and health benefits for women and children. Since then, diet has been seen as a political issue only in wartime when the government determined individual needs and rationed food rather than leaving food distribution to market forces. In consequence, as A. Oakley shows in *The Captured Womb* (Basil Blackwell, 1984), the health of women and children improved and, with the establishment of maternity services run by midwives because of the conscription of doctors, maternal and infant mortality rates declined.

Today, food chemistry is part of a major industry which offers formerly seasonal foods all the year round. Large profits are made from processed foods, often advertised and sold as snacks, which have a high 'value-added' element — crisps, for example. (You could compare the price to the farmer of unprocessed potatoes per tonne with the supermarket price of crisps per tonne.)

The twentieth century

Today, the major diet-deficiency diseases have gone — but malnutrition remains. The National Advisory Committee on Nutrition Education (NACNE) reported in 1983 that levels of health would be improved if consumption of fibre were to be increased by a quarter, sugar cut by half, fat by a third and salt by a quarter. Nutritionists point to the USA, where the rate of heart disease has gone down by 25 per cent since 1968 when people started to change their eating habits as a result of rising medical costs, public health campaigns and the Federal government's food-labelling policy.

In Britain, the Health Education Council's campaigns on diet, exercise and smoking (see Reading 7, p. 109) have been less successful. Funded by budgets which are a fraction of the total spent on advertising food, they treat diet and health as personal matters. This is a simplistic approach. Eating habits are structured by economic and social factors and influenced by the mass media.

Critics argue that the individualistic and voluntaristic approach is ineffective. Active government policy to promote healthy eating should be supported by structural measures: farm subsidies favouring vegetables and grains for human consumption rather than red meat and dairy products as at present. There should be differential pricing and advertising structures and effective labelling to help people see what they are eating. An estimated 60 per cent of our sugar comes without our knowing it in manufactured foods such as tomato ketchup, where it usually constitutes 25 per cent of the weight. So malnutrition in contemporary Britain entails both the *overconsumption* of foods of limited nutritional value and the *underconsumption* of foods necessary for good health.

The NACNE report gave a picture of 'the national diet'. For a clearer picture of *what* people actually eat and *when*, we need to look at household-based surveys. The National Food Survey documents the class and family-structure variations in diet. But its methods of data collection bias the findings towards higher income families and exclude altogether the estimated 10 per cent of meals which are eaten outside the home in school and works canteens, restaurants and chip shops. Food consumed in these settings is frequently high in salt, fat and sugar — being convenience and snack foods whose nutritional value may be limited. A case in point is the drift to 'cafeteria-style' school meals produced by rising costs, reluctant consumers and the 1980 Education Act. The Act released education authorities from the obligation to provide a third of a child's daily nutritional needs in a school dinner. For families on state benefits this may mean an absolute drop in the food value of a free school meal especially since there are no additional payments to allow parents to compensate at home for what has been left out of the school meal. Additionally, many parents, believing that the school dinner is a 'proper meal', give their children 'snack' or convenience meals when they come home.

Concern about the effects of low wages and unemployment has focused attention on the diets of the poor, the unemployed and older people. Research conducted by Manchester Polytechnic in 1984 found that the least well-nourished in their sample of different social groups were the unemployed, who frequently went without a meal in the day.

Household-based surveys, on which much of the above has been based, are criticised by Hilary Graham (*Women, Health and the Family*, Wheatsheaf, 1984) for not taking into account actual eating and distribution practices within the family. She says that food is both material and symbolic, and as such its distribution is determined by ideas about responsibility and need. Its preparation and consumption reinforce gender and domestic roles, and social relationships. It is the one area of the 'political economy of domestic life' where women can both exercise power and experience gratification. The social evaluation of family women depends on them being able to manage the housekeeping and provide 'proper meals' every day and on special occasions like Christmas in which mealtimes are the focus of social interaction. The food eaten in families is an expression of social and economic well-being, hence the significance of the 'meat-and-two-veg Sunday lunch', which may absorb as much as a quarter of a family's weekly food budget.

As she says, the table is where the poor feel their poverty most. As in Engels' day, low-income families have little choice and even less freedom where food is concerned.

Health in poor countries

Adopting a broader perspective, it has been estimated that in 1984 one-eighth of the world's population received less food than needed for survival — in fact, was starving — and 50 per cent experienced forms of malnutrition which endangered current and future health. For example, although a child may survive beyond its fifth birthday, insufficient food in infancy may hinder its physical and intellectual development: it grows up listless and susceptible to illness and parasites.

There are difficulties in mapping the extent of world hunger and illness, and the characteristics of the available data hinder the work of epidemiologists. Internationally, the resources for data collection are poor, so the World Health Organisation (WHO) and the World Bank, along with aid and relief agencies such as War on Want and Oxfam, are major sources of information. Poor countries lack the infrastructures and economic resources to collect detailed information on what is also a politically sensitive subject. Even in the rich countries where governments finance data collection it tends to be a task oriented only towards the management of existing services rather than uncovering and meeting need. In poor countries basic data on health is further limited by the fact that in many contexts no one is responsible for collecting it, and where they are, it is regarded as a bureaucratic task unconnected with the provision of health care. The information available tends to be urban-centred and aggregated and hence conceals wide variations. Still, despite these qualifications, the figures illustrate the gross disparities between the lives of people in the industrialised countries of the northern hemisphere and those of the people living in the rest of the world.

The *World Development Report* produced by the World Bank showed that in 1983 people in the world's nineteen richest countries had an average life expectancy of seventy-five years, consumed 134 per cent of their daily food requirements and had an average of one doctor for every 554 people. In the world's thirty-four poorest countries, average life expectancy was fifty years, people had 92 per cent of their daily food requirements and shared one doctor among 15 800 people. Their respective infant mortality rates were 11/1 000 and 124/1 000.

The rich countries, with 16 per cent of the world's population, have 63 per cent of total income, and the poor countries with 84 per cent have 16 per cent of total income. The USA, with 6 per cent of the world's population, has 35 per cent of its resources. In the rich world malnutrition consists of the overconsumption of too many of the wrong calories; in the poor world malnutrition means underconsumption of the right calories. Two related theories are popularly given to account for global inequalities and, although they invoke different mechanisms, both overpopulation and underdevelopment locate the reasons for Third World poverty in the countries themselves.

The WHO has argued that three measures are necessary before the health of people living in Third World countries can be improved.

1 **The provision of pure water and sewage disposal in rural and urban areas.** Water-borne infections and parasites figure prominently in the health profiles of poor countries. Most of the children under one year of age who died in 1983–84 were in poor countries; 25 per cent of them died from diarrhoeal infections and a further 25 per cent from 'childhood ailments' like measles and whooping cough, which can be fatal for the underfed.

2 **The provision of an adequate food supply.** Aside from the periodic, well-publicised famines which result in temporary increases in food aid for some areas, the vast majority of the world's population lives at levels below those recognised as being adequate for survival. As S. George has shown (*How the Other Half Dies*, Penguin, 1976), the Malthusian theory of overpopulation is often produced in explanation. Population limitation through birth control, runs the argument, would restore the proper balance between people and food supply. But in 1984, when news of the famine in Ethiopia dominated Christmas television, the world grain harvest alone was 125 per cent of total population need.

The production of surplus on this scale owes much to the Green Revolution initiated in the 1960s. Unfortunately, the high-yield strains developed were less hardy than their predecessors and brought extra costs to small-scale producers for fertiliser and pesticides. Small producers, and poor countries alike, had to borrow against future income and then generate additional income if they were to service the debts incurred.

The production of crops and primary goods for export to the West has created two kinds of vulnerability. First, indigenous food supplies may be jeopardised because the export market is seen as more profitable. Further, traditional sources of nutrition may be replaced by elements of Western diets – convenience and snack foods, fizzy drinks and milk powder for babies (see Reading 8, p. 111). Some commentators have argued that when international food and drug companies export Western life-styles, poor countries import Western diseases.

The second kind of vulnerability is that the livelihood of small-scale producers will be tied to world commodity prices. The rich countries and the large-scale producers have been the chief beneficiaries of the Green Revolution. The inequalities among countries, as well as within countries, persist. Thus the diseases of poverty can be found in countries which are net exporters of food, which have falling birth rates and rising gross national products.

According to Teresa Hayter (*The Creation of World Poverty*, Pluto, 1981), famines are wrongly called 'natural disasters'; they are a product of inequality in the distribution of food and the money to buy it. Further, power relations within and between countries mean that life for the majority of people is not being improved by what is called 'development'. In the seven largest South-east Asian countries the poor were less well off in the mid-seventies than they had been two decades before. The production of cereals – the diet of the poor – had expanded, but these cereals were consumed by the indigenous rich and people in the rich Western countries.

Teresa Hayter says that the poorest 20 per cent in Brazil get 2 per cent of the country's income; they get 3 per cent in Malaysia and 7 per cent in India. The richest 20 per cent, however, get respectively 67 per cent, 57 per cent and 49 per cent. The politics of food production and distribution between and within countries are more important than population size alone.

3 **The establishment of preventative medicine and the cheap production of 200 essential generic drugs to cure illness.** The health-care needs of the world's poor are quite different from those of the industrialised West, and yet the model of medical care preferred by governments and doctors does not recognise this (see

Reading 9, p. 111). Contrary to the view of many doctors whose training and professional self-image were gained in the West, it is argued that curative, individualised medicine is quite inappropriate. Well-equipped, prestige hospitals may enhance the reputations of health ministers among their own people and with foreign businessmen, but they do not cater for the whole population and they fail to tackle the main problems. The solution lies in programmes of immunisation and vaccination to eradicate the epidemic diseases, as in the case of smallpox, and the control of infections through sanitary reform.

The WHO has urged reform also in the ways that drugs are sold and used in Third World countries. In some parts of the world the drug bill amounts to 30 per cent of the total health-care budget (it is approximately 10 per cent in Britain). A strong argument that Western medicine is harmful as well as inappropriate is put by M. Muller in *The Health of Nations* (Pluto, 1983). He shows how the pharmaceutical industry operates differential pricing structures in poor countries, selling drugs at higher prices than in the industrial countries where they are manufactured.

All classes of drugs are promoted for conditions for which they are either ineffective or inappropriate, sold over the counter without medical supervision in countries lacking the resources to have an adequate monitoring system, and advertised in an aggressive and irresponsible way. Preparations which are banned in the West because they fail to satisfy the UK and American committees on safety are simply shipped abroad and sold in Third World countries.

In some respects patterns of illness and health in developing countries echo the changes which occurred as Britain industrialised; cancers and degenerative diseases are on the increase. But, as L. Doyal and I. Pennell show (*The Political Economy of Health*, Pluto, 1979), they coexist alongside the diseases of poverty which have largely disappeared here. They argue that there is a fundamental difference which should cause us to question the evolutionary views of health embodied in the theories of overpopulation and underdevelopment. Although standards of health rose with industrialisation in Europe, this is not the case in the poor countries of the Third World today.

4 Health inequalities

The culmination of Britain's public health reform movement came in 1948 on the centenary of the first Public Health Act with the establishment of the National Health Service. Today the NHS is the subject of considerable political debate and academic discussion concerning its ability to satisfy constantly changing health needs in society. Nevertheless, the NHS occupies a unique position in British political and social life for two reasons. First, it has the largest client group for social welfare because it provides care for people at all stages of the life-cycle; and second, more than any other welfare institution established as a result of the Beveridge Report of 1942, the NHS embodies the **welfare principle**.

The creators of the National Health Service intended that it should provide a fully comprehensive service of curative and preventative medicine for physical and mental illness. The service was to be free at the point of treatment in accordance with the patient's medically defined needs. The means-test principle of eligibility was abolished, and the service was to be funded centrally from insurance and taxation. According to one perspective, that of the first Minister of Health, Aneurin Bevan, it is 'The Jewel in Labour's Crown'. Bevan's description draws attention to the role of the Labour Party and the Labour movement in creating an institution which provides health care as a public service rather than a market commodity.

Health care prior to the NHS

By the turn of the century the occupational, status and gender divisions between and within nursing and medicine had been drawn and health services were provided on a fee-for-service basis. The system resembled a patchwork rather than an integrated service, as the extract by S. Iliffe shows (see Reading 10, p. 112). For those who could afford the premiums there were privately run insurance schemes which met some of the costs of medical treatment. Those who could not afford either premiums or fees in full might be assisted by a charity or the municipal hospitals which grew out of the asylums established after the 1867 Poor Law Act.

In 1911 the National Insurance Act established a funding system based on contributions from wages, employers and the state to pay for hospital treatment (primary health care was excluded as was dentistry and ophthalmology) for employees earning less than £160 per annum. The scheme covered about 12 million employed people: 9 million men and 3 million women. Its effects were limited because it excluded people in the middle-income ranges (just above £160), levels of benefit were low (about 10 shillings or 50 pence per week) and it operated for a limited duration. The scheme was both inadequate and inefficient:

1 it was not related to health needs;
2 its limited provisions were available to less than half the adult population at the outbreak of war in 1939;
3 it had no system in relation to the life-cycle;
4 it covered wage earners (not their dependants); and
5 it was inefficient and expensive to run because of the duplication of administrative effort by all the private insurance companies involved.

The NHS and the class structure

The political history of the foundation of the NHS tends to be written in terms of what V. Navarro calls a **power elite paradigm** (*Class Struggle, the State and Medicine*, Martin Robertson, 1976). This approach stresses the compromises to the **service ideal** which the architects of the system had to make in order to secure the involvement of key occupational groups. Aneurin Bevan's own account tells of having to 'stuff the mouths of consultants with gold' before they would agree to work in the NHS.

Navarro is critical of this type of explanation, firstly because it presents the medical sector as independent of wider political, social and economic forces. It reinforces the myth of medical neutrality and exempts doctors from political and social responsibility. If the social control dimensions of medicine were explicitly acknowledged (see Chapter 6 for further discussion), then doctors would find it hard to avoid calls for social accountability. Navarro's second criticism is that it overlooks the role of class relationships and class conflict in the evolution of social policy. Navarro himself is particularly interested in the changing characteristics of the state and the social control functions of medical health organisations.

There are three general lines in the debate about class relations and the origin of the NHS:

1 **Socialised medicine represents a victory of labour over capital**. The working class fought and won the battle for a national system of health care in the teeth of opposition from capital which gained nothing from the struggle.
2 **The NHS represents a truce in the class war**. The capitalist class had nothing to lose from the establishment of a national system of health care; indeed, capitalists gained a partial advantage because the NHS defused class conflict by providing forms of care which benefit the working class without challenging the capitalist system.
3 **The NHS operates in the interests of the capitalist class**. It has opened up new areas of economic exploitation because it is a market for the goods produced by the pharmaceutical and medical supplies industries. The costs of the service are largely borne by the working class because, although they receive the least benefit from the system, regressive taxation means they pay an increasing proportion of its costs. In addition, the lives of working-class people are regulated through medicine since it is doctors who decide who shall be exempt from responsibility and who will not. Doctors also reinforce the status quo by individualising social problems and failing to tackle their root causes.

Looking at the shape assumed by the NHS and writing very much in the social administration tradition that Navarro deplores, Honigsbaum argues that the structures established by the NHS reproduced the pre-war divisions between hospital and community medicine (F. Honigsbaum, *The Divisions in British Medicine*, RKP, 1979). He says that these divisions owed little to medical specialism or standards of excellence but a great deal to the social characteristics of patient groups and the methods by which doctors were paid. For example, there were broadly two types of hospital: first, **voluntary hospitals** which were funded in a variety of ways – by donations, endowments, fees from patients and voluntary payments such as flag days; and second, **municipal hospitals**, which were funded by local authorities empowered to charge patients what they could reasonably pay.

There were great variations in the standards of treatment and the range of services available to the population and at the same time clear indications of widespread ill health. People in low income groups were less healthy and physically smaller than people in high income groups. The associations that Chadwick had made between illness and income were confirmed by the figures for TB (increasingly regarded as a disease of poverty) showing the poor to have TB rates twice those of the rich. Comparison of health statistics within and between countries highlighted the problems. In 1939 the infant mortality rate was 42 per 1 000 live births in Surrey and 109 per 1 000 in Glasgow, which was higher than in Tokyo.

Many historians have argued that these data led to a broad political and professional consensus at the outbreak of war on the need to reform health care. As the state assumed responsibility for those aspects of social life deemed relevant to the conduct of the war, 'warfare led to welfare', in Richard Titmuss's memorable phrase. The Emergency Medical Service set up to deal with war casualties, for example, is seen as doing much to convince dissenters within the medical profession that they had little to lose and everything to gain from a national health system. Nevertheless, the consent of the medical profession, without which the system could not exist, was secured only after lengthy negotiations. Doctors were anxious that 'nationalised medicine' would turn them into salaried state employees with reduced earnings, status and professional autonomy. So they demanded and won a number of rights:

1 the right to contract out of the NHS for private medicine;
2 independence from some aspects of the NHS management structure for teaching hospitals;
3 the right of the individual practitioner to prescribe whatever treatment s/he considered appropriate (clinical autonomy); and
4 systems of payment and administration which confirmed that status differentials between hospital and general practitioners, consultants and the rest of the medical profession.

The establishment of the NHS

On the 'appointed day' (5 July 1948) all hospitals apart from the teaching hospitals were taken into the NHS to be administered by Regional Health Boards and Hospital Management Committees. Half of the hospitals acquired by the service had been built before 1891, and one in five before 1861. There were 90 000 beds in 1 142 voluntary hospitals and 390 000 beds in the municipal hospitals. The best medical facilities were concentrated in the South of England – a distribution which was perpetuated by post-war building restrictions. General practitioners provided primary medical care in association with the family-based services of local authorities, whose responsibilities were extended to include ambulance services, facilities for the elderly and services to schools.

The post-war period saw major developments in pharmaceutics and electronics which radically improved diagnosis and treatment. The modern pharmaceutical industry came into being through advances in production techniques and in therapeutic chemistry, as illustrated by the impact of the antibiotics such as penicillin. Medical practice became increasingly drug-oriented: patients judged the consultation to be successful if they left the surgery with a prescription, and doctors were faced with a growing pharmacopoeia promoted by the companies. According to some commentators (see I. Illich, Reading 11, p. 114) doctors, drug companies and the media all had vested interests in encouraging the public's belief that most conditions could be cured or controlled by 'wonder drugs'. However, there was also mounting evidence of widespread and occasionally tragic drug side-effects, and of placebo effects in drug prescribing which suggested wasted resources or trivial and unnecessary treatment (see Chapter 5).

It is not surprising, therefore, that the NHS drug bill soared, and the first stage in what many regard as the erosion of the principles on which the NHS was based came with the introduction of prescription charges in 1951. By end of the first decade of the NHS both need and cost were continuing to rise. Some post-war politicians had argued, simplistically, that the cumulative effects of the new welfare state would produce a falling demand for health care. They did not envisage the possibility of rising demand, as medical innovation offered life enhancement through new surgical and treatment techniques. The demand for spectacles, dental treatment, surgery and drugs grew. Because the cost of the service was increasingly met from taxation revenue (90 per cent in 1980) rather than from National Insurance contributions, conflicts between the Treasury and the DHSS became a feature of political discussion about the NHS.

The payment-by-capitation system in general practice had encouraged GPs in working-class areas (where the needs were great but opportunities for private practice were limited) to have long lists and correspondingly reduced time for individual patients. By the mid-1950s it was officially estimated that 80 per cent of surgeries in working-class areas occupied buildings erected before 1900, while 50 per cent of the surgeries in middle-class areas had been built after 1945.

The NHS today

Notwithstanding the improvements in health care which were achieved by the NHS, it is now the subject of many doubts. One doubt concerns the ratio of expenditure on administration to expenditure on treatment. The fact that the workforce grew between 1949 and 1979 from 400 000 to 822 000 provided ammunition for critics of the NHS, who argued that the bureaucracy was out of control and that savings in administrative services could lead to improved clinical services at no overall increase in cost. However, there is little evidence to support the contention that clinical care suffers because of administrative need. An inquiry in 1979 found that the NHS's administrative costs were the lowest in Europe (2.6 per cent of income in comparison with 10 per cent in France, for example), and it has lower bureaucratic costs than private medical schemes.

Despite rising expenditure – from 10.2 per cent of public expenditure in 1951 to 13 per cent in 1979 – substanial inequalities in the standards of treatment and care remain. Today, infant mortality is half the 1948 level but still higher than that of the Netherlands. Life expectancy has increased, but there are more workdays lost due to illness than in 1948, 45 per cent of adults have lost all of their teeth, and deaths from cancer and heart diseases have increased.

Whether or not the NHS was the product of a broad consensus, it is now a 'contested terrain' in which lay, professional and political voices debate needs and the allocation of resources to meet them. It is said that rising 'standards of living' and rising expectations in post-war Britain have produced changes in the 'need' and 'demand' for medical care. 'Need' connotes a professionally validated demand; 'demand' refers to lay-defined 'needs'. The term 'standard of living' encompasses more than personal or family disposable income; it includes access to community-provided resources or 'social goods', of which the NHS itself is an example. On the one hand, the whole concept of a 'social good' has been challenged by New Right philosophies of welfare. On the other hand, groups committed to traditional theories of welfare argue that the welfare state, and especially the NHS, has been starved of funds to the point where in many respects the system is inferior to those established by our EEC partners. The debates are grounded in political beliefs which themselves have evolved against the background of changes in post-war British social structure and in the operation of the NHS as a social institution.

Cinderella services

All Western countries have experienced a growing need for treatment of chronic conditions which require long-term medical and community care. In part this is due to ageing population structures, in part to the better life-chances of people with conditions which were once untreatable (diabetes and spina bifida, for example), and in part to the spread of conditions which cannot be cured but can to some extent be managed by careful treatment (such as cancer or AIDS).

Between 1951 and 1980 the proportion of the population in Britain over pensionable age rose from 14.5 per cent to 18 per cent and the number of people aged sixty-five and over grew from 5.9 million to 8.3 million. It has been estimated that the NHS needs to increase expenditure by 0.7 per cent per annum in real terms simply to keep pace with the rising numbers of older people in the population. Although the vast majority of elderly people live in their own homes or with relatives and are under the care of a general practitioner, the cost of providing care for those who do need hospital treatment may be high because of the nature and duration of need. In 1980, £545 was spent on hospital or community services for each person over seventy-five in comparison with the national average of £115 per person. The competition for resources between different types of need is increasingly presented in 'cost-effective' terms. One research paper into the management of financial resources published by the Royal Commission on the National Health Service (1979) described the problem as deciding to use 'substantial resources for cases where recovery can only be very limited' and deciding 'what resources should be given to prolonging the life of the very old instead of using scarce nursing and medical resources for other purposes' (p. 35).

L. Gardner in *The NHS – Your Money or Your Life* (Penguin, 1979) describes this as the **no hope, no power paradigm** in resource allocation. The clinical voice is the loudest and the most articulate. It represents organised opinion and is justified by the belief that the expertise needed to determine medical priorities rests within the profession. But two features of clinical practice – the relationship of confidence and trust between the practitioner and the patient, and the doctor's right of clinical autonomy – mean that whereas individual needs may be met, social needs may not. The resources devoted to costly techniques which currently benefit a minority of sufferers (for example, heart transplant surgery) might be better used in community or preventative medicine. But scientific and technological advance have benefited surgical rather than medical techniques and intensified the privileges of hospital medicine, which had 55 per cent of NHS resources in 1948 but 65 per cent now. The balance of power in the NHS, according to Garner, rests with the consultant groups specialising in curative rather than preventative treatment. The disparity can be illustrated by the DHSS figures (*Health Services in England, 1985*, HMSO, 1987) which show that the weekly per capita expenditure on patients in London teaching hospitals was £845.17 and in provincial non-teaching hospitals was as follows:

acute medicine	£584.53
geriatric medicine	£263.20
maternity	£687.19
psychiatric	£255.36
mental handicap	£227.01

During the last decade, a mixture of economic and medical factors has seen the rise of 'community care' as the preferred option for the elderly, the handicapped and the mentally ill, which often entails transferring people out of the NHS and into the care of bodies funded through the rates by local authorities. At a time when 'rate capping' is used as a penalty by central government to penalise 'high spending local authorities' it is obvious that community services are being financially squeezed. The client groups caught up in this situation are described by Garner as having no power themselves and no powerful medical interests ranged on their behalf because they have conditions which are not expected to be radically improved by medical advances. Today, status and career advancement go to the practitioners of high-technology medicine where scientific work holds out the hope of breakthrough. In consequence there are major inequalities in health care because of the status of the patient's condition.

Cinderella populations

There are two other forms of inequality in access to and benefit from the NHS, and to some extent they overlap with each other. Class and geographical region cut across each other – living standards and rates of employment are higher south of the Trent than in the North. Additionally, the NHS inherited a North–South division in hospitals which has not been eradicated because pre-existing provisions were augmented by post-war developments. Although governments have attempted to redress the balance by reallocating resources from privileged areas to deprived areas and by encouraging GPs, through financial incentives, to practise in poor areas, there has been very little change.

The class differences in need and in treatment are not diminishing, as the Black Report (see below, p. 47) demonstrated. Middle-class people receive more preventative treatment than do working-class people. To some extent that is a function of class differences in attitudes to illness and referral behaviour, which are the subject of the next chapter. But the middle-class also enjoys care of a higher quality: they are treated by the more experienced doctors who have shorter lists and tend to be more willing to encourage patient–doctor interaction. This has been the subject of comment by a doctor working in South Wales, an area of social deprivation, who called it the 'Inverse Care Law' (see Reading 12, p. 115).

Private medicine

During the decade since Tudor-Hart presented the Inverse Care Law there has been a growth in private medicine and a reassertion of the market principle in health care. *Social Trends* (HMSO, 1987) shows that the population covered by private schemes grew from 1.6 million people in 1966 to 4.5 million in 1985, or 8 per cent of the population. In 1982, 50 per cent of all contributions were by company purchase – in other words, they were part of group schemes provided by employers in many cases as a 'perk' to circumvent pay restraint policies. This is reflected in the socio-economic status of the people covered by private health insurance schemes – 21 per cent of men and 24 per cent of women in professional occupations, in contrast to 2 per cent of men and 1 per cent of women in unskilled manual work.

According to one view, private medical treatment is just an extension of the market principle which permits client choice at a cost. Another view is that the social significance of this expansion is rather more ideological than material. Private medicine is neither a threat nor an alternative to the NHS because it is not designed to cater for all health needs to all ages – certainly not the costly no-cure forms of health care which have low profit margins. Private medical schemes are able to flourish because of the NHS since they do not have to meet the full cost of the service provided: the training, capital, nursing and ancillary-care costs are for the most part met by the NHS.

A more critical view is taken by V. Walters (*Class Inequalities and Health Care*, Croom Helm, 1980) who argues that private medicine not only bestows an additional privilege on groups who are already socially advantaged, but it also threatens the quality of care available in the NHS because it allows high-status workers, the consultants, to divide their time between two employers, one of which is heavily subsidised by the system they undercut. It also erects another layer of disadvantage, because middle and upper-class patients benefit from both nationalised medicine and the extended benefits attached to private care. For the subscribers to private medicine it is simply a way of jumping the NHS queues for surgery. Were this group to apply political pressure for more money for the NHS rather than resolve their personal problems privately then everyone would benefit, including the old and the handicapped, who cannot opt out in the same way. Waiting lists are a major cause of patient dissatisfaction with the NHS. Between 1976 and 1985 the waiting lists grew by an average of 14.5 per cent – but in urology there were 76 per cent more people waiting to go into hospital and 40 per cent in orthopaedics. This latter group, composed largely of older patients whose lives are impaired by restricted mobility, accounts for 19 per cent of all patients on waiting lists.

The Black Report

Taking its name from the chief scientist at the DHSS who chaired the inquiry, Sir Douglas Black, this report investigated patterns of morbidity, mortality and health care in post-war Britain. It generated considerable controversy, partly on account of its recommendations and partly because of official attempts to impose limits on the circulation of the report. In the Foreword to the report, which was written by the Secretary of State for Social Services, Patrick Jenkin, two reasons were given for the government's decision not to implement the committee's recommendations: costs and doubts about the effectiveness of the proposals. In his view, the committee had failed to elucidate clearly the factors responsible for health inequalities. An edited version of the report was produced by Townsend and Davidson. Despite government rejection, the academic community accepted the report as a solid piece of research, and followed it up with a large number of studies, which are reviewed by Margaret Whitehead in *The Health Divide* (The Health Education Council, 1987).

Findings of the Black Report

1 The mortality rates of men are higher at every age than those of women, and in recent decades the relative difference has increased.
2 For men who are economically active there was a greater inequality of mortality between occupational classes I and V both in 1970–72 and 1959–63 than in 1949–53.
3 For economically active men the mortality rates of occupational class III and combined classes IV and V for

age groups over thirty-five years either deteriorated or showed little or no improvement between 1959–63 and 1970–72. Relative to the mortality rates of men in classes I and II they actually worsened.

4 For women aged 16–54 the standardised mortality ratios of combined classes IV and V deteriorated. For married and single women in class IV (the most numerous class) they deteriorated at all ages.

5 Although deaths per 1 000 live births in England and Wales have diminished among all classes, the relative excess in combined class IV and V over classes I and II increased between 1959–63 and 1970–72.

6 During a period of less than a decade, maternal mortality fell by more than a third. Although that of class I fell less sharply than the other classes, inequality between the more numerous class II and classes IV and V remained the same.

7 Among children between one and four years of age, there has been a small reduction in the class differential (especially for girls), for children aged 5–9 little or no change, but for children aged 10–14 an increase in the differential.

(P. Townsend and N. Davidson, *Inequalities in Health – the Black Report*, Penguin, 1982, p. 74–75)

The class gradient in sickness and health

Evidence of a persistent class gradient in health and sickness had been steadily accumulating since the mid-fifties, despite rising general standards. In other European countries, by contrast, standards have reached higher levels and class inequalities are diminishing. In 1960 Britain had the eighth lowest rate of infant mortality in the world, but by 1978 it had dropped to fifteenth as improvements in other non-European countries, such as Hong Kong and Singapore, overtook it. One approach to Britain's low position in the international tables of health is to argue that the very poor health of the poorest in this society depresses the statistics overall. There is only an element of truth in this since, instead of a simple break between the statistics for socio-economic class V and the rest, there is a gradient between all socio-economic groups.

The committee reviewed the evidence on health by gender, age, ethnicity, region and occupational class and found, first, patterns of unequal access to and take-up of health services, and second, 'disappointing' class gradient in life-chances that thirty years of the NHS had failed to remove (see p. 47, Findings of the Black Report).

The report's authors concluded that the significant factors affecting health were income, occupational characteristics, education, housing and life-style – all of which lie well beyond the power of the NHS to change. They reviewed in turn the four types of explanation which could be given to account for their findings, and concluded that the structural explanation was the most convincing.

1 **The artefact explanation**. According to this view, social mobility is gradually eliminating class differentials because the groups in the poorest health also belong to class V, which is a declining part of the population. Against this view it has to be said that, although declining in proportional terms, this group is increasing numerically. It is the divisions between the classes rather than any divide between class V and the rest which needs to be explained.

2 **The social selection explanation.** According to this view, which has a good deal in common with the 'natural selection' viewpoint of nineteenth-century evolutionism, people with poor health drift down into the bottom strata of society. Hence problems precede social location rather than flow from it. This argument signally fails to explain the fact that disadvantage occurs at all stages of the individual's life-cycle.

3 **The structural explanation**. Here it is structural factors lying behind the immediate control of the individual which are responsible for the patterns in health and mortality. Although the mechanisms are not fully understood, it is clear that two sets of factors play a role: **working lives** – stress, security, exposure to toxic products, shift-work and monotony; and **market position** – income, housing class, the amount of domestic comfort in the form of heating and living conditions, quality of diet and access to leisure.

4 **The life-style and culture explanation**. This view concentrates explanations for poor working-class health on such factors as

smoking, diet and inadequate exercise, but it fails to question the degree to which people's life-styles and habits reflect real choice.

Inequalities in health — conclusions

The committee made a number of far-reaching policy recommendations which concentrated on three areas:

1 improved facilities and resources for the health of mothers and children;
2 priority for disabled people to improve the quality of their lives in general, to be cared for in their own homes and to reduce the risk of their needing institutional care;
3 priority for preventative and educational action to encourage good health and discourage unhealthy habits like smoking. It had a clear set of recommendations on tobacco and cigarettes – that all advertising and sports sponsorship should be banned, that excise duty should be increased to give a price disincentive, that there should be more public no-smoking areas and more resources expended on informing people about the harmful effects of smoking as well as supporting them in their attempts to give up the habit.

The overall conclusion, however, was that without a government strategy to reduce poverty none of these recommendations would be entirely effective.

Government costing of the report's general recommendations produced a sum of £2 billion, which was deemed too costly. Costings of some of the smaller-scale proposals were not made, yet as Whitehead shows there was widespread support for the suggestions from statutory and voluntary bodies involved in caring for many of the deprived groups – the elderly, children and the handicapped – mentioned specifically in the report. Indeed, as Whitehead says, successive public opinion polls have shown the electorate in general to be increasingly in favour of government expenditure on measures to reduce health inequalities.

Although the government has accepted the World Health Organisation's policies on 'Health for all by the year 2000' the outlook is not good. The prime cause of ill health, poverty, has continued to touch more and more lives.

In 1979 a total of 11.5 million people (22 per cent of the population) were experiencing poverty; in 1981 the figure had increased to over 14 million (27.5 per cent of the population), and by 1983 it had increased again to 16.3 million (30.5 per cent of the population). (Whitehead, *The Health Divide*, p. 94)

Work, unemployment and illness

The debate about illness and socio-economic status has been given an added dimension by the continuance of high levels of unemployment. Although Durkheim's 1897 study of suicide can be seen as the first sociological enquiry into relationships between illness and economic change, research into the specific problem of illness and unemployment began with a series of studies undertaken during the inter-war depression. This tradition has been recently developed by researchers using a mixture of epidemiological and case-study methods in Britain and the USA.

The publication which had the greatest political and academic impact was M. H. Brenner's study of Britain ('Mortality and the National Economy – a Review of the Experiences of England and Wales, 1936–7', *The Lancet*, 15 Sept. 1979). He compared the indicators of economic activity over the period 1936–76 with the rates for 'social pathology' over the same period. The statistics on death, alcohol consumption, suicide, murder and admission to mental hospital all showed an upward swing within two years of a down-turn in the business cycle, and area studies showed that the increase was greatest in parts of the country most vulnerable to depression and unemployment. Brenner's statistics showed that a 1 per cent increase in unemployment was followed by a 2 per cent increase in deaths, and although he did not demonstrate the mechanism by which the effect was produced, he hypothesised that unemployment was the causal factor.

Researchers have attempted to see to what extent Brenner's findings are either statistical artefacts or ecological fallacies by conducting research into the lives of people experiencing unemployment. There are a number of issues to be explored. First, how does one explain the time-lag shown by Brenner's data? Second, how does unemployment exacerbate the already poor life-chances of socio-economic groups at the bottom of the class structure? Unemployment has a class basis, in that the risk and frequency of unemployment increase as you go down the class structure. It is in these social groups too that social deprivation even among those in work is at its greatest, so unemployment should not be bracketed off from the broader issue of poverty. What effect would a return to full employment have on the experience of deprivation? Finally, using arguments which are similar to those reviewed by the Black Report, some researchers questioned the relationship between illness and unemployment by suggesting that illness could be a factor in the decision to make an employee redundant.

The idea that unhealthy people lose their jobs first is disputed by D. S. Cook and colleagues (Health of Unemployed Middle-Aged Men in Great Britain', *The Lancet*, 15 June 1982), who showed that 18 per cent of workers who had no illnesses before losing their jobs later developed heart disease, in comparison with 9 per cent among those still in employment. The same difference (26 per cent and 15 per cent) applied to the incidence of lung diseases. Similarly, research into a 1 per cent sample of the population (see A. Sinfield, *What Unemployment Means*, Martin Robertson, 1981) found that the death rates of the unemployed were 30 per cent higher than those of the employed.

The factors accounting for the differences are given as stress coupled with loss of self-esteem and material disadvantages consequent on downward social mobility. Studies of families (see L. Fagin, *Unemployment and Health in Families*, DHSS, 1981) have shown that these effects are experienced by the whole family and not just the unemployed individual.

The experience of unemployment seems to be structured into a number of stages which correspond very closely to the social psychological concept of a **career**. The first reaction is of shock and denial, then people enter the **holiday** phase when job-loss is viewed as temporary and as an opportunity to catch up on household chores and repairs. This gives way to increasing anxiety and stress, and in the long run people accept an **unemployment identity**. At this stage they have become resigned to unemployment and engage in job-seeking in only a half-hearted fashion. L. Fagin and M. Little (*The Forsaken Families*, Penguin, 1984) found that after twelve months on the dole men, especially, mentioned health problems and seemed to be following a pattern of sick-role behaviour. Psychologists have argued that the sick role, in exempting people from responsibility, may be a more acceptable social identity than being known as unemployed.

Stress and cancer

Research into cancer shows that the unemployed have a 40 per cent greater incidence of cancer than the employed. And, since unemployment is known to be a stressful experience, this finding supports the argument that stress plays an important role in illness in general and cancer in particular (the work of Meyer and Haggerty, referred to in the next chapter, illustrates this connection for minor conditions too).

Professor Hans Eysenck, for example, has argued that cancer is caused by the interaction of psychological and physical factors – hence the fact that some people who are exposed to known carcinogenic substances do not develop cancers. In America this approach has been incorporated into a regime for cancer patients which has been pioneered by Carl and Stephanie Simonton. They encourage patients to 'visualise' the cancer and mentally fight it through images of the body's defences attacking tumours. They say that susceptibility to cancer is affected by personality type and the experience of particular life events. The following elements recur in the life-histories of their patients: the loss of an important relationship, an inability to express emotion and unresolved tensions in the patient's present relationships.

Whatever the therapeutic value of their approach, it belongs to the tradition which tends to individualise illness and place responsibility for it on the individual. In a critical review of the literature, L. Doyal (*Cancer in Britain – the Politics of Prevention*, Pluto, 1983) argues that there are two different positions in the study of cancer.

The orthodox view

Industrial process and production play a minor role. Although industrial carcinogens have been known since the link between soot and scrotal cancer was made in the nineteenth century, they account for small proportion of cancers today. The variations in cancer by individual, class and region are the result of choices people make about their life-style, smoking and diet. Into this category Doyal places the work of R. Doll and R. Peto (*The Causes of Cancer Today – Quantitative Estimates of the Avoidance Risks of Cancer in the USA Today*, Oxford, 1981), who represent the modern epidemiological tradition which, she says, acknowledges the causal significance of environmental and structural factors but presents the remedy in individualistic terms – changes in eating habits, exercise and smoking.

Doll and Peto argue that approximately 80 per cent of all cancers are avoidable, and list the following causes in their order of importance: smoking, alcohol, diet, food additives, reproductive and sexual behaviour, occupation and industrial pollution. They say that the modern life-style alone does not explain the rising cancer statistics, and that three other factors should be taken into account: now that the stigma attached to cancer is gone it is being more openly acknowledged and hence is recorded more freely; better diagnostic techniques have improved the chance of a cancer being detected and recorded; and there is an ageing population which increases the incidence of cancer.

But cancer is not a condition exclusive to older people, and despite the vast amounts of money devoted to cancer research, treatments and survival rates have not significantly improved over the last thirty years. In other areas of medicine, scientific advance usually leads to the replacement of one therapy by another, but cancer therapies accumulate. Radiotherapy began in the 1890s and was augmented in the 1940s by chemotherapy. Since then, surgical advance accounts for most of the improvements in survival rates. The five-year survival rate in 1930 was one in five, in the 1980s it is one in three simply because people survive the surgery – but die later from the cancer.

Britain has the highest rates of lung cancer in the world. There is an epidemic, according to commentators who have traced the incidence from 15 per million in 1918 to 900 per million in 1968. The link between smoking and lung cancer was established by an ingenious study which had a significant impact on the smoking habits of the medical profession. In 1950 R. Doll and A. B. Hill ('Lung Cancer in Relation to Smoking', *British Medical Journal*, 30 Sept. 1956) sent questionnaires dealing with smoking habits to all registered medical practitioners and received replies from two-thirds. Over the next five years they kept a record of all doctor deaths and compared the cause of death with the information about smoking collected by their survey. They found that death from lung cancer was positively related to cigarette consumption.

The radical view

Although it can be acknowledged that smoking and diet are important factors in the causation of cancers, they cannot be separated analytically from the economic and environmental structures of our society. Doyal (*Cancer in Britain*) argues that environmental and work-related factors play a prime role in cancers both directly, through their effects on people's health, and indirectly, because they create the needs which are satisfied by individual habits like smoking.

Cancer is preventable, but only through political and economic change. If everyone gave up smoking tomorrow cancer would not disappear because the causes of cancer lie in three areas: in work, in consumer products and in the general environment. The structures of control and protection in these areas are poor. We have limited information about the properties of substances freely used in our society. There are over 60 000 chemicals used in industry, for example, and only a fraction of them have been tested. Even where a substance has been shown to be toxic, the standards of exposure and their enforcement are limited in law to what is 'reasonably practicable'. In other words, health may be sacrificed in the interests of production; workers get compensation rather than protection and then only long after they have been able to prove conclusively that a particular substance or process was toxic. The conflicts between health and production which are taken for granted in industrial societies are illustrated by the chemical leaks at Bhopal and Seveso and the failure to enforce safety standards in asbestos production in Hebden Bridge.

The case of asbestos

1906: A Home Office report sounds the first warnings about asbestos.
1928: The first piece of government research into asbestos finds four-fifths of workers with more than twenty years' service in the industry suffering from asbestosis.
1932: Asbestos dust-control regulations were introduced – but they were unenforced, disregarded and ineffective be-

cause they permitted levels of dust above those resulting in cancer.
1935: The link with lung cancer was unequivocally established. During the thirty years that the regulations were in force there were only two prosecutions.

> The Ombudsman (whose report was published in 1976 after an inquiry requested by a former employee at Acre Mill, Hebden Bridge) ... emphasised the dangers of working with asbestos and criticised the Factory Inspectorate for failing to enforce the regulations regarding effective safety measures. Some 2 200 workers had been employed in the mill from its opening in 1939 to its eventual closure in 1970. More than 260 of these workers (12 per cent of the total) have already developed asbestos-related diseases, and, according to a local doctor, *at least 59 of those workers he could trace* had died of such diseases by 1978, 44 of them from lung cancer or mesothelioma.
> (Doyal, *Cancer in Britain*, p. 53)

The case of asbestos is illustrative of a number of issues:
– the tendency towards a litigious approach, where injury has to be proved after the event in order to receive compensation for loss of livelihood or health;
– the difficulty of establishing the agent of ill health and of tracing people who worked in the industry;
– the practice of reducing compensation to claimants who could be shown to be blameworthy, as in the case of asbestos sufferers who were also smokers – their deaths would also be recorded in such a way as to exclude the possibility of industrial disease;
– the difficulty of establishing the agent of ill health when its effects can begin to occur only after a long time lapse, even though very small exposure periods can cause irreversible damage in the long run;
– the cumulative effect upon a community where microscopic particles, carried into the home in the hair or on work clothes, can be toxic to relatives of workers;
– the fact that independent scientific expertise in support of a compensation claim is difficult to obtain since experts are likely to be in the employ of the industry itself.

5 Being ill

Sociology challenges the bio-medical model of illness which predominates in lay and professional circles. Broadly, the model rests on the following assumptions:

– that normally people are either free of symptoms of ill health or are unaware that they are ill;
– that illness consists of deviation from a set of biological norms;
– that emotional or physical changes which are biological in origin make people aware that something is wrong;
– that the initial response to something being wrong is lay remedies such as rest, an early night or perhaps a proprietary medicine;
– that if the symptoms persist or get worse people will visit the doctor;
– that at this point the person is either diagnosed as sick and treated by the doctor or assured that there is nothing wrong;
– that the person who has been diagnosed as sick follows a course of treatment prescribed to make them well at which point they are pronounced cured.

The categories of illness and disease

Acknowledging that a great deal of informal health care goes on outside of medical settings, the bio-medical model nevertheless suggests that people *normally* go to see the doctor when they have a painful or life-threatening condition which cannot be cured by self-medication.

Sickness behaviour is a concept used by sociologists to distinguish between disease (a biological category) and illness (a social category). **Disease** refers to biological states such as a fractured limb or a tubercular lung, and **illness** refers to both the subjective feeling of being unwell and the social status of **sick person**. Defined by Robinson (*The Process of Becoming Ill*, Tavistock, 1971) as 'the way in which given symptoms may be differentially perceived, evaluated and acted upon (or not acted upon) by different types of persons', the concept of sickness behaviour encompasses all of the following:

1 self-medication;
2 referral by the self or by others to lay and professional people;
3 the social dimensions of diagnosis and treatment; and
4 the characteristics of medical settings where the roles of **healer** and **patient** are performed.

Sociologists and anthropologists argue that the meanings of disease and the experience of illness are social phenomena, and they see illness not as a unitary state but as a collection of states shaped by life experiences and group values (see Reading 13, p. 116).

The relationships between biological and social phenomena

Health and illness are structured by social forces acting upon biology. As we saw with cholera and the diseases associated with poverty, malnutrition is an important factor and is itself as much a function of distribution as production. As we saw with unemployment, stress is another social phenomenon which affects health. As far as infections are concerned, peaceful coexistence seems to be the norm since we are surrounded by bacilli but we are not constantly ill.

> This observation was explored by R. J. Meyer and R. J. Haggerty ('Streptococcal Infections in Families' *Paediatrics*, vol. 29, 1962) in a year-long study of fifteen Boston families which showed how stress acted as a trigger for illness. By comparing the incidence of illness, recorded in diaries of family life kept for the project, with the presence of disease confirmed by regular throat swabs and laboratory tests, they demonstrated that biological infection is a necessary but not sufficient condition of illness. There were occasions when the levels of infection were high yet no illness was reported, and when illness was reported it tended to be during periods of family stress.

Social factors shape illness by being directly related to biological states and also by providing the vocabularies of normality and abnormality around which illness is defined. Studies of clinical interaction show that doctors' responses to patients are shaped not solely by the physical conditions presented but also by sets of socially and scientifically validated expectations. In the case of the elderly, clinical practices are informed by and in turn reinforce the widely held view that ill health is a natural consequence of ageing. The result is differential treatment regimes, allowing the elderly to suffer from treatable conditions which would not be overlooked or taken for granted in young patients for whom no medical **cost-benefit** calculation applies. It has been suggested by one writer (A. Comfort, *A Good Age*, Mitchell Beazley, 1977) that three-quarters of the infirmities commonly associated with old age are socially rather than biologically produced.

The bio-medical model presents lay and folk remedies as the base of a pyramid of health care which has scientific-specialist medicine at its apex. The doctor's role is to discover the cause of the ailment and provide an effective remedy at the same time as dispensing reassurance and advice to the patient. Here the link between the physical condition, or disease, and the **social status of the sick person** is clearly defined and bound by the assumption of rationality. According to the model, abnormal or irrational behaviour can be attributed to patients who either consult their doctors for trivial conditions or who fail to refer the 'symptom iceberg' of serious conditions.

Trivial consultations

Research by A. Cartwright and R. Anderson (*General Practice Revisited*, Tavistock, 1981) has shown trivial consultations to be a significant element in doctors' lack of job satisfaction. Comparisons of general practice in 1968 and 1977 found that, despite considerable improvements in many respects of medical work (investment in appliances and buildings, reductions in out-of-hours and night-visiting and increases in ancillary support), doctors had neither higher levels of job satisfaction nor better relationships with patients.

Patients tended to dislike the changes in clinic management and organisation which had taken place between 1968 and 1977 because they felt separated from doctors by such gatekeepers as medical receptionists. Younger doctors practising **whole-person medicine** who had dispensed with the more rigid versions of the bio-medical model were found to have the highest levels of job satisfaction. Job dissatisfaction was associated with a lack of interest in psychiatric approaches in general practice and, although the reasons given for liking the job had changed over the period in question, the reasons for disliking it had not. The same proportions in 1968 and 1977, a quarter of all GPs, felt that half of all consultations were for trivial, time-wasting complaints. One half also felt that patients did not respect them enough. Many doctors felt that patients had a growing tendency to refer with medically irrelevant problems related to domestic difficulties.

Trivia are dismissed by doctors because they may implicate factors beyond their professional competence, yet there is a strong suggestion, in the work of Meyer and Haggerty (above), for example, that trivia may be important factors in the onset of illness.

Social skills in medicine

Discussions of trivia implicate two different models of medicine – medicine as a science and medicine as an art. The latter is seen to be most appropriate to general practice because it emphasises the social skills involved in consultation. Here, in private discussion of uncertain and intimate aspects of life, doctors have to depend more on the information given by patients than on their own abilities to detect and interpret physical symptoms (see Reading 14, p. 117).

The management and treatment of illness clearly involve more than the application of scientific knowledge in formal settings. Furthermore, changes in the pattern of illness have accentuated the importance of the social concomitants of illness. Alongside the technical and scientific aspects of medicine there are psychological and counselling dimensions which may all be differently ranked by the participants.

Prescriptions and placebos

Research into aspects of clinical practices, such as repeat prescriptions (M. Balint, *Treatment or Diagnosis*, Tavistock, 1970), reveals that doctors sometimes play a part in initiating the very conduct for which they criticise their patients. For some patients the doctor *is* the medicine. In these cases no causal relationship exists between the treatment and any subsequent improvements in health. There is, rather, a **placebo effect** involving two factors:

1 the self-limiting nature of the condition, meaning that it will heal or disappear in due course with the proper diet and environment; and
2 the influence of mind over matter either because the problem has an emotional root which will respond to reassurance or because the body's immunities will be stimulated by feelings of well-being and anxiety reduction.

In these cases, therefore, the repeat prescription is less a treatment for illness and more a diagnosis of the doctor–patient relationship. Repeat prescriptions can be a coping mechanism initiated by doctors for time-consuming and frustrating cases which involve a string of recurrent symptoms for which no rational therapy or satisfactory diagnosis exists. The symptoms are a product of unhappiness with life, not physical disorder. Balint's colleagues discovered that patients resisted change once started on such treatments, even though the drugs were pharmacologically irrelevant. These conclusions are supported by R. E. A. Mapes (*Prescribing Practice and Drug Usage*, Croom Helm, 1980), in which 32 per cent of long-term repeat prescriptions were for psychotropic drugs and 30 per cent were for ill-defined conditions such as nervousness.

Prescriptions have a symbolic significance representing a successful consultation to both parties in general practice. But studies of how patients actually use their prescribed treatments show that one-fifth of pills are not taken as advised. The reasons for this include: feeling better and so the tablets are unnecessary, fear of 'getting hooked' and generally disliking pills. Additionally, those who take the pills may do so in therapeutically ineffective ways and tolerate worrying side effects which go unreported. Professionals tend to view behaviour of this kind, **non-compliance**, as irrational and puzzling (M. E. J. Wadsworth *et al.*, *Health and Sickness*, Tavistock, 1973), but for sociologists the real puzzle is compliance. Part of the answer resides in doctor–patient role relationships and in the status position of the doctor described by Balint as 'the medicine called doctor'. Professional and lay expectations that the doctor will be able 'to do something about it' constrain doctors to act. This may involve prescribing drugs which mask other problems. It is clear that doctors are not always willing actors in the process of **medicalising social problems**. As the rise in prescriptions for psychotropic drugs shows, there are three important factors:

1 People are presenting problems which lend themselves to psychological interpretations — symptom for symptom, women's problems tend to be interpreted as psychological and men's as organic (see Reading 15, p. 118).
2 Some symptoms are clearly related to **problems of living** and the emotional demands of looking after other people. Studies of mothers, especially lone mothers, reveal high levels of social and material deprivation and stress. Men have more material and political resources than women and a wider range of culturally acceptable coping mechanisms. Alcohol is an acceptable outlet for men, which is freely available outside of the medical control structures governing the distribution of tranquillisers — women's functional equivalent.
3 The co-operation of patients and carers is necessary for the management of the largest growing category of disease — chronic illness. And co-operation depends on knowledge, symptom control and stress reduction — often through drugs.

Symptom iceberg

Turning to the other type of abnormal behaviour identified by the bio-medical model, why are many serious conditions not referred to doctors? It was found as long ago as 1954 in Peckham that only 40 per cent of those who felt ill visited the surgery and, more recently, that less than 25 per cent of troubling complaints tend to be referred. Sociological research shows that the vast majority of illness symptoms are never referred for professional help; that feeling healthy and feeling well have little to do with the absence of physical symptoms, since illness and health are related to the social values of the group.

Community studies have proved to be very valuable in addressing some of the issues raised by the 'symptom iceberg': concepts of health and illness, practices of self-referral, the relationship between lay, folk and professional systems of healing, access to and distribution of health services and the class gradient in the use, as well as provision, of services (see discussion of the Black Report in Chapter 4, p. 47). Jocelyn Cornwell's research in Bethnal Green (*Hard Earned Lives*, Tavistock, 1984), for example, looked at communication among kin, friends and the statutory services and at the ways in which people evaluate various specialisms. Maternity, for example, was seen as a common-sense rather than scientific enterprise, and so doctors involved in this area were accorded less deference than other specialists and judged by different criteria — expressive criteria such as 'manner' rather than instrumental criteria such as technical expertise. M. Blaxter and E. Paterson (*Mothers and Daughters*, Heinemann, 1982), in their study of three generations of working-class women, found that they viewed illness fatalistically as largely a matter of luck. They were also far less willing to visit the doctor than doctors believed them to be.

In a study on a larger scale and involving interviews conducted in 1 344 households registered with one general practice (D. R. Hannay et al., *The Symptoms Iceberg*, RKP, 1979), 70 per cent of respondents thought themselves to be in perfect or good health and 22 per cent described themselves as fair. Neverthless, one-third were taking medicines (mostly sedatives) and one-third had at least one serious medical symptom causing severe pain. In 25 per cent of cases the pain was severe enough to cause inconvenience. The majority had done nothing about their symptoms apart from, in 15 per cent of cases, having general discussions with the family. The symptoms iceberg turned out to be 2.5 times the rate of trivial consultation and was closely related to social problems. The authors expressed their concern about the high levels of very serious unreported symptoms — blood in phlegm and in faeces, for example — and they suggested that doctors should reconsider the 'trivial consultations' concept. Medical mannerisms, clinic organisation and posters advising people with 'flu symptoms' to stay at home may be discouraging the wrong people from visiting the surgery.

The reasons given for failing to see the doctor about worrying symptoms include not wanting to trouble the doctor, being discouraged by the waiting room, the appointment system or the receptionist, fearing that the doctor will adopt a judgmental attitude and hoping that the problem will go away.

In summary, the link between feeling ill and becoming a patient is a tenuous one, and defining oneself as ill need not result in readiness to consult a doctor. The question framed by the biomedical perspective — 'Why do people delay going to the doctor?' — has been rephrased by sociologists as 'Why do people go to the doctor in the first place?'

The decision to go to the doctor

According to I. K. Zola (*'Pathways to the Doctor — from Person to Patient'*, Social Science and Medicine, 7, 1973, 677—89), there are a number of triggers sanctioning professional help:

1 the effects of the symptoms upon the sufferer's interpersonal circumstances and how they are perceived by people close to the sufferer;
2 the extent to which the symptoms interfere with a valued social activity;
3 the degree to which the sufferer comes under social pressure to 'do something about it' — in introducing the symptoms to the doctor people often justify coming by referring to family pressure;
4 the nature and quality of the symptoms.

In respect of the last trigger, empirical studies have produced contradictory findings. Some (Hannay, Robinson, *op. cit.*) have found no clear-cut relationship between the clinical severity of symptoms and their presentation to the doctor, although others have (Wadsworth, *op. cit.*). These differences in findings may result from the definitions of 'severity' used. Wadsworth's research also found no class gradient in consulting behaviour even though inter-class communication barriers have been a feature of research in the area ever since Hollinshead and Redlich examined the influence of class on diagnosis of mental illness in 1958 (see Chapter 6).

David Mechanic (*Medical Sociology – a Selective View*, Free Press New York, 1968) has suggested two other factors which may influence referral behaviour:

1 the possession of a vocabulary to symbolise and express the distress experienced; and
2 the cultural and situational constraints affecting the expression of distress.

Comparison of Jewish, Italian, Irish and 'Old American' patients in New York revealed different ways of expressing and understanding pain (M. Zborowski, 'Cultural Comparisons in Response to Pain', *Journal of Social Issues*, vol. 16, No. 8, 1952). The white, middle-class 'Old Americans' were stoical in their approach to pain, the Irish denied pain, the Italians sought pain relief and the Jewish-Americans were concerned about the pathology underlying the pain.

Research in a community in South Wales (D. Robinson, *The Process of Becoming Ill*, RKP, 1971) revealed that neither the severity of symptoms nor the type of disorder led people to the doctor. Using 'sickness diaries' kept by twenty-four families, information about consulting behaviour and normative information gained from discussion of hypothetical sickness situations, Robinson found that the major factors in referral behaviour are ideas about (1) occupational demands, (2) illness, (3) the inconvenience of the medical system, and (4) the perceived dangers and threats involved in treatment in relation to the danger of the illness.

He discovered inequalities of access to the status sick which was not guaranteed by even professional validation and severe symptoms. The meaning of physical symptoms varied with the age, gender and socio-economic status of the sufferer. Tiredness, quietness and irritability, for instance, were regarded as symptoms of illness by women and middle-class people in general but not by working-class men. A class consensus existed around performance of occupational role as a major priority, and people were not seen as 'deserving ill' if they could accommodate the symptoms to that role.

The sick role

Research in this area has been heavily influenced by Talcott Parsons' writings on the sick role (*The Social System*, RKP, 1970). Located in a structural functionalist account of medicine in industrial societies, it is described as a socially sanctioned form of deviancy possessing the following characteristics:

1 the sick person is exempted from normal social responsibilities;
2 the sick person cannot be expected to look after herself;
3 the sick person is expected to desire a return to normality; and so
4 the sick person is expected to seek competent professional help.

Because sickness interferes with normal social responsibilities and permits exemption from them, it may be resorted to by people unwilling to meet their social obligations. Consequently, in addition to its therapeutic function, medicine monitors and promotes an awareness of social obligation among the sick.

At the inter-personal level, Parsons sees the doctor–patient relationship as symmetrical; patient vulnerability is protected by expertise and a code of ethics. The doctor's position of trust and responsibility, requiring a long training period and high ethical standards, is policed by professional associations and rewarded by high social and economic standing.

The concept has generated a good deal of criticism on empirical and theoretical grounds. First, the model conflates the sick role and the patient role, although it is possible to have one without the other. Second, the social control function of medicine makes medical neutrality an impossibility. Third, the image of mutuality and reciprocity in Parsons' model assumes a correspondence of interest between the participants which is denied by empirical evidence of conflict in doctor–patient interaction. Fourth, the ideals of high ethical standards and community service are ideological constructs legitimising medical power. And fifth, illness cannot be seen as a form of deviance because it is governed by social norms (see Reading 16, p. 119).

A model devised by Szasz and Hollander to cater for the variations from Parsons' model found in empirical studies described three types of therapeutic relationship depending on the nature of the medical problem and the treatment location:

1 **activity/passivity**, where the doctor is the dominant actor, as in the case of emergencies and many surgical operations;
2 **co-operation/guidance**, where the patient co-operates with medical advice, as in Parsons' classic formulation; and
3 **mutual participation**, where, as in the case of allergies, psychotherapy and so on, patient and practitioner work together and, as with chronic illness, where self-care is essential for the management of the condition.

For logical completeness, though not empirical accuracy, according to E. Freidson (*The Profession of Medicine*, Harper & Row, 1979) there are two other possibilities:

4 **guidance and co-operation** in which the doctor plays a submissive role; and

5 a relationship in which the **patient is active and the doctor is passive**.

Freidson argues that ambivalence and conflict are central features of doctor—patient interaction because of such structural and cultural features as power differentials. The characteristic of functional autonomy (clinical freedom) in medical work distinguishes it from other classes of occupations and allows doctors to act largely independently of lay and peer evaluation.

The routines of medical work

Medical work is a set of day-to-day activities as well as a set of structural relationships, and the Parsonian paradigm overlooks the bargaining, negotiation and exchange of communication which are part of the enterprise. Some researchers (such as G. Stimson and B. Webb, *Going to See the Doctor*, RKP, 1975) have made this issue the focus of their work, using Goffman's concept of the **encounter** or focused interaction:

1 the encounter is fixed in time and space;
2 it is specific in its focus (help and advice are being sought) and specific in the forms of talk and interaction permitted; and
3 there is a competence gap between the participants.

Going to the GP was not the immediate solution to uncertainty, as problems were initially aired in informal settings in which small talk about health is part of routine social interaction. Here, and later on in the waiting room, the 'story' of the symptoms was constructed and rehearsed before its official telling in the surgery. How the story would be told was carefully planned, especially in cases where the doctor was a gatekeeper to other services which the patient required. Patients prepared their part in the consultation and anticipated the various contingencies which could arise during it. It was not always immediately clear whether or not the consultation had been successful in producing the expected outcome, so it was evaluated and assessed later. An example is the discovery at the pharmacy that the same 'useless tablets' have been prescribed again!

Often the consultation was discussed in conversation with other people, and at this point another kind of 'story', a medical 'horror story', was told. These accounts were at variance with the observations actually made by the researchers who had attended the consultations. Stimson and Webb were interested in the form of these stories — usually dramatic eye-witness accounts depicting the patient as active, more knowledgeable than the doctor and making categoric statements. Derogatory language and unflattering nicknames for the doctor featured very prominently. So did descriptions directly opposed to the conventional view of the profession — laziness, incompetence, unworldliness and self-interest. The worst atrocity stories were usually counterbalanced by tales of exemplary medical conduct. This medical gossip was regarded as a strategy to restore the power imbalance between doctors and patients.

According to Freidson, control of the patient and control of information are essential parts of the medical process. But control is not easily won since patients are not passively involved, as J. A. Roth showed in his study of tuberculosis patients (*Timetables*, Bobbs-Merrill, 1963).

Staff in the sanatorium tended to individualise TB and discourage patients from making comparisons with one another. They failed to provide information as readily as patients demanded it, either because there was little progress to report or because the uncertainty of progress without remission made it unwise to raise a patient's hopes. Patients reacted by seeking information about their condition and stage in the disease process, and by informally exchanging information they constructed informal theories about the normal course of the disease. 'Getting better' was indicated by a series of treatment stages or **benchmarks**. This form of common sense was the background to bargaining with staff on discharge or transferral to the next stage in the treatment process.

Communication

Concern about information has also been explored as a general feature of hospital life. A. Cartwright (*Human Relations and Hospital Care*, RKP, 1964) says that going into hospital means entering a large-scale institution at a time when the patient is most vulnerable and least able to comprehend his surroundings. To some degree, all of the patients she interviewed experienced the mortification of self which Goffman argues is a defining feature of total institutions (see Chapter 6), and 60 per cent mentioned lack of communication as a problem — either in being unable to frame the right questions or in not getting answers with enough detail. There were no class variations in this respect, though there were in the degree of distress and domestic disturbance caused by going into hospital and in also in the likelihood of a visit to the hospital by the GP (4 per cent of working-class patients and 14 per cent of middle-class patients).

The main source of information for patients was the doctor (46 per cent), then the sister (28 per cent), the nurse (11 per cent) and other patients (2 per cent). Patients were conscious of the social and occupational distance between themselves and the medical staff (only 7 per cent of doctors introduced themselves to patients), and they felt that doctors failed to understand their feelings and needs. This was especially true for surgical staff, with whom two-thirds of patients had not discussed their anxieties even though they had seen the surgeon before entering hospital. More information about their medical treatment was wanted by 12 per cent and 23 per cent wanted information about their nursing care. The information desired ranged over a large number of issues and the need for it was felt at different times, but patients did not feel they ever had the unhurried atmosphere and intimacy necessary to ask questions. Although nursing staff could be an important source of information they were limited first by what they had a right to communicate to patients and in what detail, and second by the risk that talking to patients would interfere with other ward duties (see Reading 18, p. 121).

Cartwright concluded that bureaucracy might not actually achieve its objective of ensuring the delivery of good health care since the information collected on a patient is diffused by a large number of people — all specialist practitioners — who do not communicate directly with one another and therefore could not adopt a holistic approach to the patient.

Medical strategies and coping mechanisms

Ways in which patients turn to their advantages what Cartwright regards as organisational deficiencies are given in Strong's research (P. M. Strong, *The Ceremonial Order of the Clinic*, RKP, 1979). With each new clinical consultation the doctor compiles a case history from the patient, who is thus given the opportunity to re-tell her story with a different emphasis or inflection. Nevertheless, patient autonomy is limited by the high levels of control exercised by doctors through such procedures as the following:

1 **Inhibitory routines**, which limit the patient's influence on the treatment process. Two examples illustrate this point:
 (a) Studies of cancer experiences show that doctors defer unwelcome treatment decisions until 'after tests', at which point the patient feels either unable or unqualified to be involved in the decision process;
 (b) In paediatrics doctors may bypass normal conventions and address the child directly when they wish to limit parental influence or opposition to recommended treatments.
2 **Reactive routines**, which reduce the involvement of the patient by failing to divulge the medical options which have been considered and rejected. Doctors often use forms of speech which effectively close discussion.
3 **Reconciliatory routines** designed to accommodate patients to treatments which they are known to reject. Doctors exploit the medical division of labour and bureaucratic structures to avoid confronting the patient with unwelcome information. They can transfer responsibility for decisions — to operate, for example — to another practitioner or specialist. Bad news can be communicated to patients via letters to the GP who inherits the patient's objections or concerns.

The use of these routines as medical coping mechanisms as well as control mechanisms has been explored by studies of chronic and degenerative illness in which communication is either the main form of treatment or the pathway to palliative care. A case study (B. Glaser and A. L. Strauss, *Anguish — the Study of a Dying Trajectory*, Robertson, 1977) of terminal illness in hospital examines these points in some detail. Staff responsible for the care of a woman dying of cancer, Mrs Abel, were uncomfortable with her response to her condition and their own reactions to the manner of her dying. They lacked an institutional structure through which the issues raised by terminal care could be confronted and resolved in a manner supportive of staff and patient. As a consequence, they began to avoid her and delegated responsibility for her care to marginal staff members — part-timers and trainees. At the time of her greatest need, therefore, she experienced progressive social isolation and no continuity of care. Glaser and Strauss point out that the organisation of hospital work meant that no one was responsible for checking that she had been given the information she wanted; no one was responsible for overviewing the quality of her care; and there was no one to prepare her for death.

Medical typifications

For a variety of reasons Mrs Abel was regarded as a 'bad patient', and her case illustrates the way in which medical treatments are affected by professional typifications of 'good' and 'bad' patients.

A study of how medical students become doctors (H. S. Becker et al., *Boys in White — Student Culture in the Medical School*, University of Chicago Press, 1968) traced the origin of some of these typifications. In this study good patients were people whose conditions provided interesting or useful case notes. 'Crocks' were cases of no instrumental value to medical students because they either had routine ailments or ailments with a disorganised pattern of symptoms or because the patient could not or would not talk about the condition in such a way as to facilitate diagnosis. Rose Coser's study of patients in a Jewish hospital in New York (*Life on the Ward*, Michigan State University Press 1962) showed 'bad patients' to be people who failed to give a good account of their symptoms or who, in giving their account, affronted the doctor's self-esteem — speaking in Yiddish rather than American English, for example. Patients also develop typifications of good and bad doctors according to their evaluation of the expressive and technical dimensions of medical practice.

Much of this empirical work suggests an **invisible pedagogy** in which the patient has to be flexible in her conduct towards the doctor and be prepared to switch roles at different stages in the interaction process. A. Schutz's typology of relationships to knowledge (*On Phenomenology and Social Relations*, University of Chicago, 1970) is relevant in this connection. He describes three relationships towards specialist knowledge: expert, well-informed citizen and 'man in the street'. In the terms of the bio-medical model, rational behaviour demands that the patient should be like the well-informed citizen and know when it is appropriate to seek expert help. However, once in the consulting room the patient must revert to the status of the 'man in the street' and surrender all knowledge and responsibility to the professional. In other words, the sick person is encouraged to participate in the therapeutic process but the patient is excluded from it.

6 Social control and medicine

The idea that medicine is an important institution of social regulation in modern societies is expressed by the **medicalisation of society** thesis. In its simplest formulation, the thesis does not relate medicine to other institutions and refers to it as though it were a unitary profession. Thus it ignores the consequences of (1) divisions by specialism and (2) competition for resources. Nevertheless, it does focus attention on the ideological and practical consequences of the growth of medicine as an institution (see P. Strong, *The Ceremonial Order of the Clinic*), and encourages us to explore the nature, source and beneficiaries of medical power.

According to the thesis, medicine is part of the ideological state apparatuses of modern societies. Not only is it a means of social regulation, but it also gives a science a human face, which legitimises its economic and political power. That we may all have had occasion to benefit from aspects of medical care (despite its horror stories and mistakes) blinds us to the dangers of scientific and medical imperialism. One exponent of this view (Illich, Reading 11, p. 114) describes medicine as a 'sickening' force in society. Others claim that we have become dependent upon medicine to solve problems of living and have surrendered moral responsibility to an occupational group only too willing to take it over. Thomas Szasz (*Ceremonial Chemistry*, RKP, 1974), for example, argues that medical values and rituals have replaced religious ones, and doctors, no more than competent technicians of the body-machine, have assumed the mantle of a 'secular priesthood' possessing, like their medieval counterpart, a moral monopoly. More recently, Ian Kennedy's Reith Lectures on power and responsibility in modern medicine argued that ethical issues posed by such 'medical advances' as 'test-tube' reproduction and experimental medicine are either going by default or left to doctors to resolve.

Some of the issues raised by the thesis — medical power and autonomy, and ideology and science — have been addressed in sociological research into two, often related areas, **mental illness** and **women's health**.

Mental illness

On the continuum of theories about mental illness there are two polar opposites which are rooted in different theories of the person.

> *Polarised models of mental illness*
>
> BIOLOGY AND MENTAL ILLNESS AS ORGANIC DISORDER
>
> Insanity is in fact disorder of brain producing disorder of mind; or to define its nature in greater detail, it is a disorder of the supreme nerve-centres of the brain — the special organs of the mind — producing derangement of thought, feeling and action, together or separately, of such degree or kind as to incapacitate the individual for the relations of life.
> H. Maudsley, *Responsibility in Mental Disease*, Kegan Paul, 1906, p. 11–12)
>
> ANTI-PSYCHIATRY AND THE MYTH OF MENTAL ILLNESS
>
> The term 'mental illness' is a metaphor. Bodily illness stands in the same relation to mental illness as a defective television set stands to a bad television programme. Of course the word 'sick' is often used metaphorically. We call jokes 'sick', economies 'sick', sometimes even the world is 'sick', but only when we call minds 'sick' do we systematically and strategically misinterpret metaphor for fact — and send for the doctor to cure the 'illness'! It is as if a television viewer were to send for a TV repairman because he dislikes the programmes he sees on the screen.
> (Thomas Szasz, 'Bad Habits Are Not Diseases', *The Lancet*, ii, 128, 1972, p. 84)

Although most practitioners in the field of mental illness do not wholly subscribe to Maudsley's formulation, and acknowledge that social processes have some influence, these are not incorporated into the theories which concentrate upon genetic, bio-chemical and psychological factors within the individual. The social systems within which the individual is located are not central. Such approaches tend to emphasise the physical dimensions of mental illness and favour physical treatments such as drugs, surgery or Electro-Convulsive Therapy (ECT). Evidence that personality changes, mood swings and behavioural disorder can all be linked to physical factors such as brain damage, chemical imbalance and allergies provides ample justification for this approach. Additionally, the fact that physical measures can regulate symptoms and produce the feeling of progress which comes slowly from time-consuming and exhausting sessions of 'talk-based' therapies makes them attractive. So, although social factors may be regarded as relevant to cause, diagnosis or treatment they are not seen as central to the phenomenon itself. Consider the following:

1 What does the association between behavioural disorders such as 'hyper-activity' in young children and allergies to food additives, such as the orange colouring tartrazine, suggest about the significance of the food cultures of different age group?
2 What inferences may be drawn from a report on ECT in the September 1987 *Bulletin of the Royal College of Psychiatrists*? It mentioned that between 1980 and 1984 ECT administrations dropped by 17 per cent, from 150 000 to 125 000. Awareness of its negative public image and opposition from social workers and nurses made doctors reluctant to use it even though *they* believed it to be effective against depressive disorders.

Although not going as far as Szasz, many writers have developed approaches to mental illness which are based on social processes and address such questions as: 'what are the contingencies leading to the diagnosis of mental illness? What personal and social consequences follow the diagnosis? and What is the significance of conformist and non-conformist behaviour in the phenomenon?

Patterns in the distribution of mental illness

The fact that there are patterns in the distribution of mental illness and cultural variations in the experience of suffering and disorder provide justification for an investigation into the social forces acting upon the person. The nature of those forces and the mechanisms involved in the 'production' of mental illness are matters for debate, and so there are a number of theories whose principal

All hospital admissions, 1984

Percentage admissions of men and women by age group

	55–64 yrs	65–74 yrs	75+ yrs
Male	38	36	30
Female	62	64	70
	100	100	100

Age/sex specific rates

	55–64 yrs	65–74 yrs	75+ yrs
Male	93	146	402
Female	116	176	421

At all ages women are more likely to be hospitalised than men.

Women constituted 66 per cent of patients admitted for senility, 67 per cent of those admitted for treatment for depressive illness (29 per cent of all people admitted to psychiatric institutions were for treatment of depressive disorders), but women were 31 per cent of those who were admitted for treatment for alcohol dependency, alcohol psychosis and alcohol abuse.

Men were 41 per cent and women 55 per cent of in-patients in all types of psychiatric institutions including hospitals with child and adolescent psychiatric beds.

Source: In-patient statistics from *The Mental Health Inquiry for England for 1982*, HMSO, 1985

difference is the degree to which they accept the 'reality' of mental illness and conventional medical categories.

Thomas Szasz

Szasz believes that there is no such thing as mental illness and that the parallels with physical illness suggested by the terminology are erroneous. There being neither consensus nor clarity in medical accounts of its causes, symptoms and effective treatments, the key element in any theory of mental illness is the **social characteristics** of patient and therapist. A study conducted in New York (D. L. Rosenhan, 'On Being Sane in Insane Places', *Science*, 179, 1973, p. 250–58) provides uncomfortable support for this position. Eight 'sane' people (**pseudopatients**) gained admission to twelve different hospitals by complaining of hearing voices. Apart from changing their names and occupations they told no other falsehoods and conducted themselves 'normally'. In all but one case they were diagnosed on the basis of a single symptom as schizophrenic. The rule of caution, leading to false-positive diagnoses, and the routines of neglect in psychiatric institutions can explain the failure of professional staff to detect their sanity despite the accusations of inmates that the pseudopatients were 'not crazy'. There were interesting developments following the disclosure of the research when the pseudopatients left hospital after an average stay of nineteen days (the range was seven to fifty-two days). The cases of 193 patients, none of whom was connected with the project, were reviewed by the authorities and forty-one were confidently diagnosed as 'sane-pseudopatients' by one or more members of staff!

Szasz sees mental illness as a euphemism for unhappiness or deviance, and therapy as a reclassification process absolving people from normal social obligations. He believes that psychiatric techniques can enhance self-knowledge, but not in their present institutional form. Institutional psychiatry permits authorised groups to persecute deviants and lay people to evade the problems of life by playing risky games such as 'nervous breakdown' or 'hysteric'.

His views are close to those expressed by Andrew Scull in *Museums of Madness* (Penguin, 1979), that the emergence of psychiatry and the spread of lunatic asylums in the early nineteenth century were not liberal and scientific advances in the understanding of insanity. They were, rather, part of the new systems of classification and regulation developed during industrialisation to deal with problem urban populations.

Thomas Scheff

Scheff analyses mental illness as a social construct through six key concepts: norms, rule breaking, deviance, role, career and labelling.

In *Being Mentally Ill* (Aldine, 1966), he examines the ways in which an act of deviance may lead to the acquisition of a deviant identity — **mad** (corresponding to Lemert's primary and secondary deviance). He says that many social rules become visible through their infringement but that rule-breaking usually goes unnoticed much of the time either because it is transitory or people make the adjustments necessary to cope with it. When people break rules it is for a variety of reasons and deviant conduct is either denied or accepted as a facet of the person — as eccentricity. Occasionally it provokes a response, and the mad game' is initiated. This game is easily played, because its rules are generally known through the stereotyped images of madness learned early in childhood and reinforced by popular culture. Being 'mad' means 'acting crazy' and 'not knowing that there is something wrong'. Getting better depends upon acknowledging that 'there is something wrong'! One is punished for denying the role and rewarded for accepting it. One does not become mentally ill through mysterious physical processes; rather, one takes on the mad role in circumstances structured according to social norms. It is a coercive process because it occurs at a time of crisis when the person is highly suggestible, and it offers as the only viable option a stigmatised role which alters the person's social identity and self-image in ways that have consequences for their future participation in society.

Scheff's contribution to a theory of mental illness has been to emphasise the conditions under which the transgression of normative boundaries leads to labelling. In common with Lemert, he presents the medical profession as participants in a moral enterprise who are authorised to validate social norms, apply the label 'mentally ill' and make it stick (see Reading 20, p. 123).

Erving Goffman

Goffman takes the patients' viewpoint and uses the concept of **career** — an ordered series of status transitions — to describe their experiences. He says that the starting point is forms of deviance which others perceive as warranting complaint and intervention. The pre-patient is asked to account for their actions by people with a legal or other mandate to sanction treatment and committal. The support of kin and other relations is reduced or even withdrawn altogether as kin and officials act in alliance against the person. The pre-patient stage ends in feelings of abandonment, betrayal and confusion which are compounded by the depersonalisation and mortification rituals which the patient undergoes on admission to the mental hospital. Here the person is re-socialised into a new (**stigmatised**) status and a new culture (the hospital), through the removal of the person's former identity along with the symbols and rights which supported it. Now an object of other people's actions rather that a subject in his own right, the patient has to learn and accommodate to the rules of a **total institution**. This he describes as a 'forcing house for new identities', because it is an enclosed community where all aspects of life are closely regulated and erstwhile rights are regarded as privileges. Total institutions are characterised by great social distance between the staff and inmates, who develop hostile and contradictory points of view and come to perceive each other in narrow and stereotypical ways. The psychological survival of patients depends upon alternative sources of meaning and status via the inmate subculture.

Although Goffman's work has stimulated considerable discussion it has also elicited criticism for being overdeterministic, like a novel, and unempirical. The coercive picture drawn by Goffman is inconsistent with the fact that most mental patients are out-patient, most are voluntary patients and many people have been successfully treated for childhood disorders and adult neuroses and compulsions without acquiring the disabling stigma he describes.

R. D. Laing

Superficially, Laing and Szasz have much in common: both are qualified psychiatrists who turned a critical eye upon their profession; and both have stimulated new approaches to mental illness when their ideas became popularly known during the 1960s. Unlike Szasz, however, Laing believes that mental illness is a reality whose origins and nature have been misunderstood because of the presumption of irrationality. He contends that the symptoms of mental illness are the only form of communication available to people experiencing fundamental and disorienting crises of identity. Therapists should listen seriously to patients because what they communicate verbally and through the metaphorical content of their symptoms renders their abnormality both intelligible and rational.

In *The Divided Self* (Penguin, 1965), he says that **schizophrenia**, one of the most baffling and common syndromes, grows out of socially generated conflicts within the self. The self is composed of two parts: the real or true self, and the imaginary self or the vision of the self as it is understood by other people. Situations in which people are required to deny their real self and present a false self which is more in tune with the expectations of others Laing describes as **schizoid** or **schizo-genic**. When a person's social network consists primarily of schizoid relationships, then the self actually fragments and the classic symptoms of schizophrenia ensue. Mental breakdown is thus a rational response to impossible demands. Laing's basic point is that our personal sense of individual security depends upon our relationships with other people and congruence between our self-image and the expectations of others.

Through his casework Laing has examined the forms of regulation and control associated with the strong emotions of love and guilt found in close interpersonal relationships. He concludes that when we are bound to other people — in the family, for instance — we strive to please them and meet expectations which may be unrealistic and a threat to our own psychological integrity.

A simplistic reading of Laing results in two mistaken beliefs: first, that he is blaming the family, parents in particular, for mental illness; and second, that he is anti-psychiatry.

Like Szasz, he values the insights that psychiatric methods produce and wants to see changes in the forms of psychiatric and therapeutic practice. Laing's work has shown that the experiential dimensions of mental illness and the 'maddening' aspects of negative imagery have a legitimate place in academic debate. He has also championed the rights of mentally ill people to be taken seriously and given the support and understanding their anguish demands.

Explanations for the distribution of mental illness

What none of the authors reviewed so far have accomplished is a theoretical explanation for the distributional pattern of mental illness. In British society, there are comparatively high levels for lower-class people against upper-class, for people of Afro-Caribbean origin against people belonging to other ethnic groups, and for women against men.

Empirical studies which have addressed these issues present explanations that can be divided into three broad types:

1 **social stress** – that some groups in society are more at risk of developing physical and mental disorders because stress is socially structured;
2 **social residue** – that people with mental disorders tend to drift down the social structure because of their illness and thereby have a concentration of disadvantage characteristics; and
3 **differential diagnosis** – that medicine is influenced by ideologies of normality which give privileges to some groups and control others – for example, the sexual double standard excuses 'sowing wild oats' as normal for males but views 'promiscuity' as a symptom of 'nymphomania' in girls.

Social class

Research by A. Hollinshead and F. Redlich in New Haven in the 1950s (*Social Class and Mental Illness*, Chapman Hall, 1958) reported class differentials in diagnosis. The lower down the social scale a person was the higher their chance of being diagnosed as psychotic – seriously ill and dangerous.

The follow-up in the mid-1970s uncovered a reduced class differential in diagnosis but a persistent differential in treatment. Practitioners generally advocated psychotherapeutic approaches but actually used them infrequently with lower-class patients. Examination of treatment regimes showed treatment status as mirroring social status. Lower-class patients had less frequent contact with doctors who were more likely than not to be juniors.

Ethnicity

Examining the relationships between ethnicity and mental illness, R. Littlewood and M. Lipsedge (*Aliens and Alienists, Ethnic Minorities and Psychiatry*, Penguin, 1982) remark that British citizens of Afro-Caribbean origin

1 have high rates of diagnosed schizophrenia,
2 show a greater likelihood of being an involuntary patient,
3 are more likely to see a junior doctor; and
4 are more likely to have ECT or powerful psychotropic drugs than other groups in the population.

Admission rates to hospitals per 100 000 people over 15 years of age standardised to accommodate the different age structures of the different ethnic groups

	Country of origin: England & Wales	Scotland	W. Indies	India	Pakistan
Schizophrenia					
Male	87	90	290	141	158
Female	87	97	323	140	103
Manic depressive psychoses					
Male	45	42	30	31	22
Female	92	99	31	57	38
Neuroses					
Male	48	56	19	33	36
Female	88	111	67	64	103
Personality disorders					
Male	43	100	27	36	18
Female	41	67	46	29	55

Source: Adapted from R. Cochrane, 'Mental illness in immigrants to England and Wales: an analysis of hospital admissions, 1977', *Social Psychiatry*, 12, 24–35 – *A Comparative Study of Mental Illness among Immigrant and Native People*

They say that the treatment situation would be improved if there were more therapists drawn from ethnic minority groups and a greater commitment on the part of psychiatrists to working with people from ethnic minorities. These steps might ensure that help-seeking behaviour occurs at an early stage and leads to ways of offering therapy which reduce cultural taboos on the expression of emotions to strangers.

As to causal factors, it is accepted that migration may be a factor in some cases since migrant populations are heterogeneous and include rootless and vulnerable individuals. Additionally, in Britain the stress of migration has been compounded by racial discrimination and harassment. This is probably the most important cause of the high rates of mental illness for native Britons of Afro-Caribbean origin. The language of distress is affected by culture, situation and reaction to the negative stereotyping which is experienced by young men in particular (for example Rastafarians). Clearly, racism also affects diagnosis and treatment since, as we have seen, doctors are not immune to the political and moral prejudices which structure our social typifications.

The large proportion of inmates in secure psychiatric institutions who are Afro-Caribbean is an index of a basic social rule: if you belong to a 'problem group' you will be subject to high levels of social regulation generally. In the case of psychiatric disorder, the degree of official intervention depends upon two factors which initially may not be related: severity of symptoms and status of the patient.

Gender

Rates of mental illness, calculated by whatever measure, are higher for women than men. It is the only area of deviance (perhaps with the exception of prostitution) where women outnumber men. According to one theoretical approach this is not surprising, since female deviance tends to be viewed as illness in any case. So do women actually experience more mental disorders than men, and if so why? Are the differences simply an artefact of gender expectations — doctors being more willing to diagnose and women more willing to accept the diagnosis? Explanations for the phenomenon implicate three sets of factors.

1 Femininity

There are two 'common-sense' views on women and mental illness. One is that the biology of reproduction makes them more prone to mental illness than men. The other is that mental illness follows women's attempts to depart from the role mapped out for them by nature. Paradoxically, studies of post-natal syndrome have shown that women who conform most closely to the 'traditional' feminine role run the greatest risk of developing mental illness.

A stronger argument holds that femininity is not a natural expression of biological identity but a status which women achieve only by being moulded physically and psychologically according to the standards of the day. Femininity embodies contradictory ideals which are difficult to meet and devalued in relation to masculinity. As Susan Browmiller says (*Femininity*, Paladin, 1986), the effort women expend on 'being feminine' artificially accentuates the differences between women and men and allows the latter to appear 'masculine' effortlessly. Women striving to achieve the feminine ideals of marriage and motherhood battle with the stress of reality and the conventional, acceptable expression of their alienation is mental illness.

2 Women's status

Apart from any congruity between illness and femininity, it is argued that the statistics reflect the relationships women have to society's caring roles. One view is that women's problems are more readily presented and treated because they have greater access to professional help through their roles as carers, in private and public, for other people. Another, almost contradictory view, is that the well-being of women is dependent upon that of the people for whom they are responsible. They develop a heightened sensitivity to the needs of others at the expense of their own, and seek professional help on their own behalf only when they are 'unable to cope' anymore. 'People work' is a source of both satisfaction and frustration for women. Their salaried work is poorly paid and their unpaid work is held in low esteem and receives little community support. The burden of caring for dependent relatives, as J. Finch and D. Groves show (*A Labour of Love*, RKP, 1983), is often solely borne. It limits the women's opportunities for personal development and leads to illness and social isolation. Because to admit to unhappiness seems like betrayal, many emotional and psychiatric disorders go unreported.

In general, mental illness is associated with low status, lack of material possessions and lack of power. Consequently, the relationships between mental illness and marital status are interesting to note: rates are higher for married women than married men, but lower for single women than single men. This suggests that, issues of masculinity/femininity aside, marriage confers benefits on men at the expense of women.

3 The functional equivalence thesis

This thesis holds that women and men have differential access to deviant conduct. Women's lives are more regulated, both informally and formally, than are men's. Examples of this are commonsense notions of what is risky or unfeminine conduct – hanging around on street corners, for example – and the formal regulation of the workplace where women occupy roles which are often subject to male authority and allow little freedom of movement or association without permission. Another dimension of regulation is gendered ways of coping with stress. In accordance with social expectations, women internalise their frustration, whereas men can vent their feelings through acceptable activities such as aggressive and competitive sport or they can externalise their frustration through deviance.

Turning the argument about 'female expressiveness' on its head, this thesis has a number of attractive features. It suggests that male disorders, regarded as more threatening than female disorders, end up in the crime statistics rather than in the mental illness statistics. It connects masculinity to criminality and sees one as the natural consequence of the other – male sex drives and rape being the classic example. It also accommodates the fact that, on the whole, women convicted of similar offences to men receive stiffer sentences and the paradox that, although femininity may drive you mad, you will be punished if you reject it!

The thesis is problematic, however, because it generates a series of questions it does not answer. To what degree are criminality and mental illness connected? Do men and women experience similar levels of stress and frustration? How do official perceptions of male and female deviance affect the official records? What part is played by structural factors rather than individual motivations? For example, might not the high treatment rates of women for mental illness be influenced by structural factors of the same order as those which produce large female hospital populations? Women outnumber men in hospitals, first because of the institutionalisation of many aspects of women's lives (such as childbirth) which brings women under professional scrutiny. Second, the preponderance of women in the very old age group accounts for the large numbers of women in institutions. Third, conventional differences between the ages of husbands and wives which, allied to their social roles, means that sick women stay in hospitals but their male equivalents are cared for at home in 'community care'.

Empirical research by D. Goldberg and P. Huxley (*Mental Illness in the Community*, Tavistock, 1980) shows that although women figure more prominently than men in the stages of consultation and diagnosis, they are less likely to be referred to a psychiatrist and admitted as an in-patient. This suggests that the female excess in hospitals is a very small reflection of the much larger excess of mental illness they experience in the community in general.

Research by G. Brown and T. Harris in Camberwell (*The Social Origins of Depression*, Tavistock, 1978) confirms this proposition. Charting the incidence of clinical depression among patients registered with one general practice, they were surprised to find an iceberg of untreated symptoms which was almost exclusively female. Detailed analysis of the lives of 600 women demonstrated that the onset depression was triggered by specific **stressful events** such as the loss of a job, divorce or a death in the family but only in the presence of the following **vulnerability factors**: having lost her mother (not father) before the age of eleven years, having school-age children at home, lack of waged work, poor housing conditions, social isolation and the absence of a close and confiding relationship with a friend, husband or lover. It is a feature of many family lives that relationships between the spouses deteriorate after the birth of the first child and do not improve until children grow up. The vulnerability factors produce low self-esteem which, when coupled with lack of material resources, explains why some women become depressed and overwhelmed by a sense of hopelessness in life. The people most likely to suffer in this way therefore are working-class women who are full-time housewives with children under six years of age.

Medical power

It is difficult to think of another profession enjoying the same ideological, social and economic status as medicine. In 1858 the state confirmed the profession's monopoly in the labour market with the Medical Registration Act, and during the ensuing century medical perspectives have become a significant element in everyday forms of thought. As such, medicine was involved in the process identified by Jurgen Habermas as **modernisation**. He argues that, in addition to the transformation of productive relationships, modernisation entails a process of rationalisation through which traditional forms of legitimation, based on faith are replaced by legitimations or forms of explanation and justifications based on science. To the degree that medical perspectives form part of the common culture and ideological orthodoxy of all industrial societies, medicine is a powerful institution.

Today, medicine still depends upon state patronage since it is practised almost entirely within an institution funded by the state – the NHS. However, the medical profession enjoys a degree of autonomy from the state which is unparalleled by other professions in the state's employ because of its claim to expert knowledge and its commanding political position. It has gained control over the structures of health care within the NHS, which it jealously guards, as is shown by the experiences of ministers for Health trying to import cost–benefit accounting systems from manufacturing industry into the NHS.

In recent years the profession, rather than the consumer, has been at the forefront of political debate about expenditure and cuts in the health service – a development which perhaps supports Freidson's argument that medicine exercises its power primarily in its own interests. Nevertheless, at the time of writing, the medical profession is also voicing criticism of government because of the social and health consequences of its policies on unemployment. The Assistant Editor of the *British Medical Journal* reviewed government statistics on death and disease among unemployed men, and concluded that even the most cautious analysis shows that unemployed men were twice as likely to commit suicide as the rest of the population and 75 per cent more likely to die of lung cancer: 'Forty thousand are going to die prematurely before the end of the century unless we do something dramatic about unemployment' (Dr R. Smith, *Unemployment and Health*, Oxford University Press, 1987).

Expressed in its simple form, the argument that medicine acts as an agent of social control operating in the interests of society (simple functionalism) or the state (simple Marxism) is difficult to sustain. A slightly more sophisticated formulation, acknowledging relative autonomy and popular ideological support, has it that the dynamics of medical practice disguises the elements of control and self-interest. The reform of the sick note system illustrates this **relative autonomy**.

The claim that it was time-wasting and the desire to establish professional distance from the role of state functionary led to medical support for reform. Under the new system introduced in 1982, people are able to certify themselves as unfit for work if they are absent for fewer than seven days. However, since sickness benefit did not become payable until the fourth consecutive day of illness and then only on production of a doctor's certificate, the doctor's ultimate role as the 'medical police' has not been fundamentally changed. The power to confer the status 'sick' still resides with the profession, and it is held accountable by employers and the state for the responsible discharge of this function. To the observation that the offer of a personal, confidential service to people in need masks the structural causes of illness and the interests served by those structures, the profession replies that it did not cause the conditions it treats and its first duty is to the patient.

Conclusion

Stimulated by four interrelated developments, there has been a growing debate about health and medicine in popular and academic circles. They are consumerism, the limits to medicine, the resurgence of alternative and complementary therapies, and the self-help movement.

1 **Consumerism**. A characteristic of contemporary society, consumerism is implicated in demands for democratic accountability, a consumer voice in a range of services and the freedom to pay for the service one requires, whether it is private conventional medicine or less orthodox alternatives such as herbal remedies or aromatherapy.

2 **The limits to medicine**. Changes in the age structure and in the patterns of illness have meant that the bio-medical curative model is becoming inappropriate to many contemporary ills. The multiple pathologies of old age, Aids and cancer have all re-focused attention on alternative therapies as well as preventative care.

3 **The resurgence of alternative and complementary therapies**. Modelled on holistic principles, the therapies of meditation, biofeedback, massage, homoeopathy and chiropractic, to name a few, are seen as both a threat and a challenge to conventional medicine. To some degree the profession has been able to isolate the threat by undercutting some as 'mumbo-jumbo' and incorporating others under their professional regulation in 'the interests of patients'. However, the free market principle and

government support for private health care may assist the spread of therapeutic alternatives.

4 **The self-help movement**. Over the last twenty years there has been a self-help trend and growth in individual consciousness about health which has challenged professional institutions – Well Women Clinics in America are a case in point. It is interesting to note that in Britain there has been a good deal of support for such clinics, although under the NHS umbrella, which perpetuates the old client – professional relationship.

This chapter will end by voicing some reservations about the concept of 'medicalisation' and warn against adopting an overdeterministic view of the power of the institution and the social control dimensions of medical practice.

The assertion that, as medicine expanded, scientific and rational perspectives became the common currency in ideas can be challenged. Some of the studies referred to earlier show that commonsense and non-scientific approaches are still to be found in social and medical practice (for example, Balint's work on medical euphemisms and placebos). Medicine has always been presented as an art as well as a science, and the empiric approach – 'try it and see' – has an established place. Consultations between professionals and patients are covered by the conventions of politeness, clinical freedom and confidentially, which offer opportunities not only to negotiate treatments but also to practise clinical heterodoxy. As patients are not slow to notice (including the women of a certain maternity ward who had their gin and chicken takeaways smuggled in during visiting hours), in even the most tightly regulated settings there are spaces through which group and individual autonomy can be expressed.

PART 3
Statistical data and documentary readings

7 Statistical data

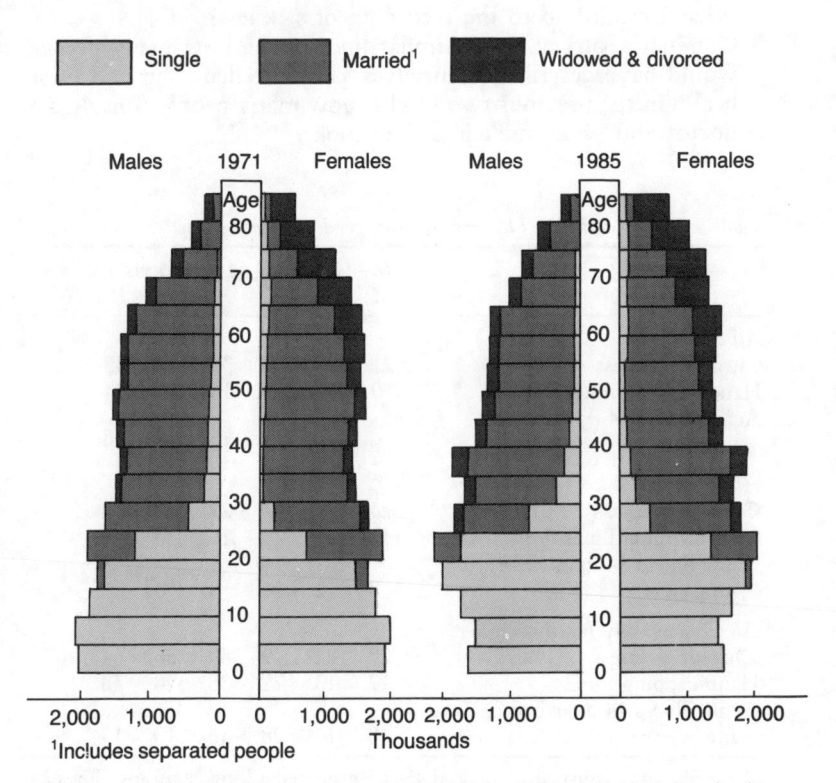

Figure 7.1 Population: by sex, age and marital status, 1971 and 1985 (England and Wales)

Source: Office of Population Censuses and Surveys, *Social Trends*, Vol. 17, HMSO 1987

Figure 7.1 shows how the population structure changed between 1971 and 1985.

Consider what implications the changes have for (1) planning the health service, and (2) the availability of 'informal' or community care.

Tables 7.1, 7.2 and 7.3 are drawn from the *General Household Survey* and they allow us to look at rates of reported sickness by gender, age and occupational status.

1 Is it possible to identify groups of people from these data who are particularly sick?
2 What factors lead to the recording of sickness?
3 Conduct a survey along similar lines to see how many people would have described themselves as in excellent, fair and poor health in the previous two weeks, how many people consulted a doctor and what medicines they took.

Table 7.1 Reported illness by employment, gender and age group

	16–44 yrs M	16–44 yrs F	45–64 yrs M	45–64 yrs F	65 yrs and over M	65 yrs and over F
All employed						
Chronic sickness	21	19	35	34	37	45
Handicapping illness	9	11	19	18	16	24
Acute illness 14 days before interview	8	11	9	12	10	9
All unemployed						
Chronic sickness	24	21	42	29	1	2
Handicapping illness	15	11	28	16	0	1
Acute illness 14 days before interview	8	12	11	8	0	1
All Economically Inactive						
Chronic sickness	28	22	79	49	56	64
Handicapping illness	17	13	72	35	40	48
Acute illness 14 days before interview	10	11	28	16	13	19

(i.e. 35% of employed men aged 45–65 reported a long-standing illness in comparison with 42% of unemployed men of the same age)

Source: adapted from the *General Household Survey 1981*, HMSO 1983

Table 7.2 Reported illness by gender and age group

	0–4 years M F	5–14 years M F	15–44 years M F	45–64 years M F	65–74 years M F	74+ M F	All ages M F
% of males and females by age group reporting chronic illness	12 7	17 13	22 21	40 41	51 58	60 70	28 30
% of males and females by age group reporting limiting chronic illness	3 3	8 6	10 11	26 26	35 41	44 56	16 19
% of males and females by age group reporting acute illness in the period 14 days before interview	13 12	12 11	8 11	12 13	11 17	15 21	11 13
% of males and females by age group consulting a GP in the period 14 days before interview	21 17	8 9	7 15* 12	13 13	13 16	17 20	10 14
Average number of days restricted through illness a year per person	17 15	14 12	13 18	26 27	29 42	48 55	— —

* 1 in 8 GP consultations for this group were related to pregnancy, childbirth and contraception.
Source: adapted from the *General Household Survey 1981*, HMSO 1983

Table 7.3 Reported illness by gender and economic activity status

	Professional		Employers & managers		Intermediate & junior non-manual		Skilled non-manual & self-employed professionals		Semi-skilled manual & personal service		Unskilled manual		All persons	
	M	F	M	F	M	F	M	F	M	F	M	F	M	F
% consulting a GP in the period 14 days before interview	8	12	9	12	10	13	10	15	12	15	12	15	10	14
% reporting long-standing chronic illness	22	18	26	26	27	28	29	28	32	36	32	46	28	30
% reporting limiting long-standing illness	10	10	14	15	14	17	16	17	20	24	19	31	16	19
% reporting acute illness in the period 14 days before interview	9	12	9	12	11	13	11	12	12	14	12	17	11	13

(ie. 12% of men employed as unskilled manual workers consulted a GP in the period 14 days before the interview in comparison with 8% of men employed as professional workers.)
Source: adapted from the *General Household Survey 1981*, HMSO, 1983

Table 7.4 Household income and individual food consumption in oz per person per week: Great Britain, 1980

	Gross weekly income of head of household		One adult, one or more children (oz)	Two adults, one child (oz)	Two adults, two children (oz)
	£67–110	Over £250			
Milk	4	4	4	4	4
Cheese	4	5	3	4	4
Beef, veal, mutton, lamb & pork	16	23	11	18	13
Poultry and other meat products	20	17	20	20	18
Fresh vegetables (not potatoes)	27	36	21	26	22
Fresh fruit	18	32	17	21	19
White bread	24	12	23	22	20
Potatoes	45	36	37	41	39
Sugar	12	8	12	10	9

Source: Ministry of Agriculture, Fisheries and Food (1982) Household Food Consumption and Expenditure, 1980, Table 20, pp. 104–6, Table 23, pp. 114–16

Table 7.5 Spending on main food items in families with children: Great Britain, 1981

	(A) Household income		(B) Household composition	
	One man, one woman and two children: gross normal weekly income of household Under £120 £	One man, one woman and two children: gross normal weekly income of household £250 or more £	One adult, two or more children £	One man, one woman and two children £
Milk	2.61	3.15	2.23	2.86
Poultry and undefined meat	2.36	2.92	2.16	2.74
Beef, veal, mutton, lamb	2.11	4.05	1.75	2.75
Bread	1.61	1.54	1.42	1.63
Vegetables (not potatoes)	1.59	2.02	1.54	1.78
Biscuits and cakes	1.42	1.96	1.38	1.83
Potatoes	1.21	1.18	1.23	1.26
Fruit	1.09	2.07	1.15	1.53
Sweets and chocolates	0.92	1.25	0.77	1.10
Total food expenditure	28.30	41.51	25.93	34.42

Table 7.6 *Meal times on supplementary benefit: meals eaten by a sample of patients and their children on the day of or the day before the interview: England and Scotland, 1980*

Children's meals				Adults' meals			
Breakfast	Lunch	Tea	Supper	Breakfast	Lunch	Tea	Supper
Cereal, eggs, toast	School dinner or sausage and beans	Rice and fish	Hot chocolate, biscuits	Nothing	Toast, coffee	Rice and fish	Milk, biscuits
Cereal	Pie & chips	Nothing	Bread & butter	Tea	Fish & chips	Nothing	*Father:* boiled egg & tea
Toast & tea	School dinner or soup & yogurt	Sausage, egg & chips	Toast & tea	Tea	Nothing	*Mother:* sandwich; *Father:* sausage, egg & chips	
Cereal & toast	Fish fingers & potatoes	Soup	Beans on toast	Drink	Soup	Drink	Drink
Cereal	School dinner	Nothing	Egg salad	Nothing	Nothing	Nothing	Egg salad
Cereal	School dinner	Spaghetti	Tea & sandwich	Coffee	Egg & toast	Spaghetti	Tea
Cereal	Beans on toast	Sausage & chips	Nothing	Nothing	Tea & biscuit	Nothing	Nothing
Cereal				Tea & toast		Tea & toast	Nothing

Source: Burghes, L. *Living from Hand to Mouth*, 1980, p. 34

96 Statistical data and documentary readings

Tables 7.4, 7.5 and 7.6 present data on food consumed in households according to income, family size and source of financial support.

1 Identify the groups having the most and least healthy diets.
2 Do Engels' observations on the diets and consumption patterns

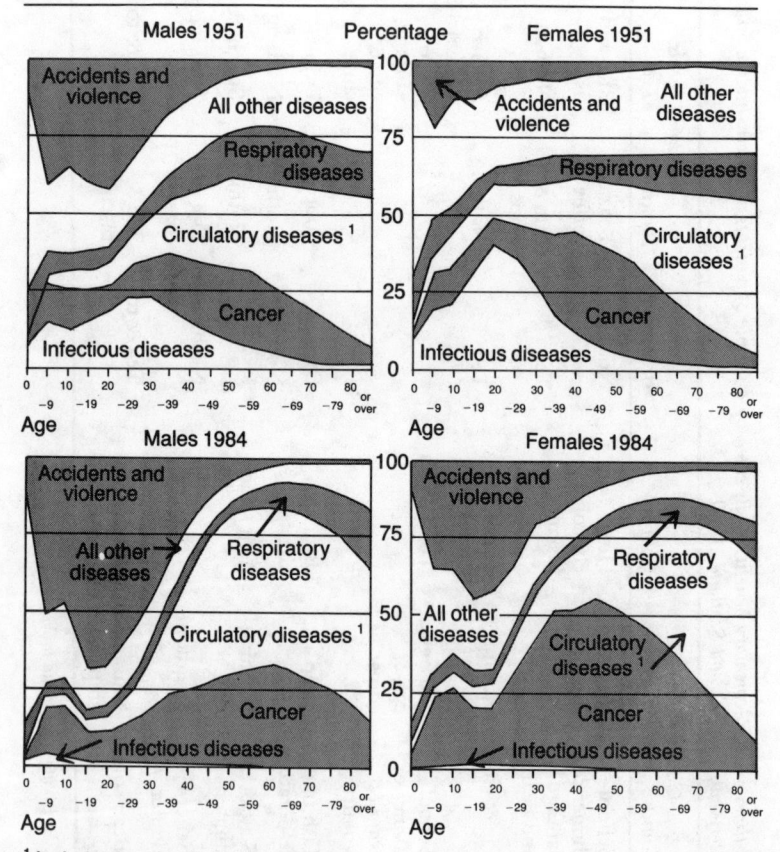

Figure 7.2 Selected causes of death: by sex and age, 1951 and 1984, United Kingdom

[1] Includes heart attacks and strokes

Source: Office of Population Censuses and Surveys; General Register Office (Scotland); General Register Office (Northern Ireland)

of the working class in nineteenth-century Salford have any relevance today? One body of opinion holds that people need education to promote healthy eating. Another view is that people are generally aware of what constitutes a healthy diet but are unable to provide it.

Figure 7.2 is rather difficult to read, but it should give answers to the following:

1 What information does it yield on the rank order of causes of death by age group, 1951 and 1981?
2 What are the chief differences in the two periods by gender?
3 What support do the statistics give for life-style theories of illness?

Table 7.7 Causes of death, 1959–69

	1959	1961	1963	1965	1967	1969
TB						
Male	228	191	170	123	108	76
Female	214	188	142	121	115	68
Cervical cancer						
Female	110	106	104	102	101	99
Heart disease						
Male	173	159	142	117	103	100
Female	181	171	150	118	101	96
Appendicitis						
Male	220	180	146	134	106	96
Female	166	170	149	133	107	96
Breast cancer						
Male	83	106	91	102	113	99
Female	92	96	97	97	101	103
Venous thrombosis & embolism						
Male	57	69	82	87	100	103
Female	56	70	83	87	96	104
Cirrhosis of liver						
Male	91	106	99	100	92	105
Female	94	98	93	96	96	109

Source: Standardised Mortality Ratios (1968 = 100) for selected causes of death in England and Wales, adapted from A. L. Cochrane, *Effectiveness and efficiency*, Nuffield, 1972

It is suggested that the decline in mortality produced by the reduction in infections has been negated by increases in degenerative conditions.

1 For which conditions are the differences between men and women greater than the similarities?
2 Do the figures suggest that our common assumptions that breast cancer is a female complaint and heart attack a male complaint should be altered?

Table 7.8 *Smoking behaviour among secondary school children: by sex and school year, 1984, England and Wales, percentages and numbers*

	Boys					
	1st year	2nd year	3rd year	4th year	5th year	All years
Percentage who:						
Have never smoked	75	52	41	32	23	44
Tried smoking once	17	28	25	28	22	24
Used to smoke	4	10	9	14	14	11
Smoke occasionally	4	7	12	10	10	9
Smoke regularly	0	3	12	17	31	13
Sample size (= 100%) (numbers)	332	396	409	392	395	1,928

	Girls					
	1st year	2nd year	3rd year	4th year	5th year	All years
Percentage who:						
Have never smoked	76	55	48	30	25	46
Tried smoking once	16	26	22	23	21	22
Used to smoke	3	9	9	13	14	10
Smoke occasionally	4	8	12	9	11	9
Smoke regularly	1	2	9	24	28	13
Sample size (= 100%) (numbers)	305	364	338	341	340	1,689

Source: *Smoking among secondary school children in 1984*, Table 2.7, J. Dobbs and A. Marsh, Office of Population Censuses and Surveys

Table 7.9 Adult cigarette smoking: by sex and age, Great Britain, percentages and numbers

	Age group						All persons	Average weekly cigarette consumption per smoker
	16–19	20–24	25–34	35–49	50–59	60 or over		
Percentage smoking cigarettes								
Males								
1972	43	55	56	55	54	47	52	120
1976	39	47	48	50	49	40	46	129
1980	32	44	47	45	47	36	42	124
1982	31	41	40	40	42	33	38	121
1984	29	40	40	39	39	30	36	115
1984 Sample size (numbers)	672	789	1,572	2,116	1,170	2,098	8,417	
Females								
1972	39	48	49	48	47	25	41	87
1976	34	45	43	45	46	24	38	101
1980	32	40	44	43	44	24	37	102
1982	30	40	37	38	40	23	33	98
1984	32	36	36	36	39	23	32	96
1984 Sample size (numbers)	671	855	1,745	2,351	1,289	2,877	9,788	

Table 7.10 Prevalence of cigarette smoking among persons aged 16 and over* by sex and socio-economic group, Great Britain, 1972 to 1980

Socio-economic group	% smoking cigarettes				
	1972	1974	1976	1978	1980
Males					
Professional	33	29	25	25	21
Employers and managers	44	46	38	37	35
Intermediate and junior non-manual	45	45	40	38	35
Skilled manual and own account non-professional	57	56	51	49	48
Semi-skilled manual and personal services	57	56	53	53	49
Unskilled manual	64	61	58	60	57
Total	52	51	46	45	42
Females					
Professional	33	25	28	23	21
Employers and managers	38	38	35	33	33
Intermediate and junior non-manual	38	38	36	33	34
Skilled manual and own account non-professional	47	46	42	42	43
Semi-skilled manual and personal service	42	43	41	41	39
Unskilled manual	42	43	38	41	41
Total	42	41	38	37	37

* Aged 15 and over in 1972.
Source: OPCS, Monitor, *General Household Survey 1981*

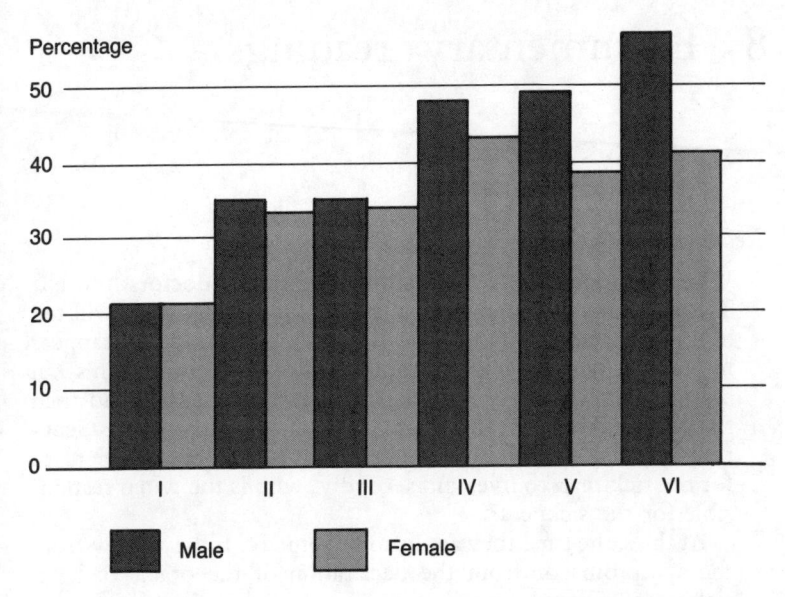

Figure 7.3 Prevalence of cigarette smoking among persons 16+ by sex and socio-economic group, 1980

Source: *General Household Survey 1981*, HMSO, 1983

From Tables 7.8, 7.9 and 7.10 and Figure 7.3 you should be able to say which groups in the population are more likely to smoke and which groups are more likely to give up smoking.

1 Why do people take up smoking, and why do they find it hard to give it up?
2 Conduct a survey to see how many people under the age of sixteen can correctly identify the cigarette brands associated with sponsored sports.

8 Documentary readings

Reading 1   Magic and medicine

When a Zande suffers from a mild ailment he doctors himself. There are always older men of his kin or vicinity who will tell him of a suitable drug to take. If his ailment does not disappear he visits a witchdoctor. In more serious sickness a man's kin consult without delay first the rubbing-board oracle and then the poison oracle, or, if they are poor, the termites oracle. Generally they ask two questions — firstly, where is there a safe place for the sick man to live, and secondly, who is the witch responsible for the sickness?

At the same time they apply some remedy. If they know from the symptoms or from the declaration of the oracle that the sickness is caused by good or bad magic, a specialist who knows the antidote is sent for without delay, and he administers a drug specific to the magic. If the sickness is due to witchcraft they combine efforts to persuade the witch to leave the patient in peace with the administration of drugs to treat the actual symptoms of the disease. . . . No treatment, however, will prove efficacious if a witch is still attacking the sick man and vice versa, the treatment is sure to be successful if the witch withdraws his influence.

(E. E. Evans-Pritchard, *Witchcraft, Oracles and Magic among the Azande*, Oxford University Press, 1937, pp. 588–89)

Questions and activities

1 Describe the differences in personnel, training, treatment methods and relationship of healer to sick person between modern medicine and any other form of healing.
2 In what respects might scientific and magical approaches to sickness and healing be distinguished from each other?
3 Compile a list of the common remedies recommended for colds, flu, hiccups, stomach upset and headaches.

Reading 2 The plague

In France: reaction to the onset of plague in 1322 took the form of revived anti-Semitism and Jews were accused of causing the black death by poisoning the wells. They were persecuted and burned and driven eastwards.

In Italy: Such was the energy of the contagion of the said pestilence that it was not merely propagated from man to man, but, what is much more startling, it was frequently observed that things that had belonged to one sick or dead of the disease, if touched by some other living creature, not of the human species, were the occasion not merely of sickening but of an almost instantaneous death. Whereof my own eyes had cognisance, one day among others, by the following experience. The rags of a poor man who had died of the disease being strewn about the open street, two hogs came thither, and after, as is their wont, no little trifling with their snouts, took the rags between their teeth and tossed them to and fro about their chaps; whereupon, almost immediately, they gave a few turns and fell down dead as if by poison, upon the rags which in an evil hour they had disturbed.

(G. Boccaccio (trans. J. M. Rigg), *The Decameron*, Dent, 1968, p. 6)

Boccaccio tells us that in 1348 people responded to the plague in one of three ways: first, by 'living temperately and avoiding every kind of luxury'; second, by 'drinking freely, frequent(ing) places of public resort and tak(ing) their pleasure with song and revel' and mocking the plague; and third, by deserting the city and fleeing to the country (the choice he made himself).

In England: However, the poor people could not lay up provisions, and there was a necessity that they must go to the market to buy, and others to send their servants or their children; and as this was a necessity which renewed itself daily, it brought abundance of unsound people to the markets, and a great many that went thither brought death home with them. . . . It is true that people used all possible precaution. When anyone bought a joint of meat in the market they would not take it off the butcher's hand, but took it off the hooks themselves. On the other hand, the butcher would not touch the money, but have it put into a pot full of vinegar which he kept for that purpose.

... He never used any preservative against the infection other than holding garlic and rue in his mouth, and smoking tobacco. And his wife's remedy was washing her head in vinegar, and sprinkling her head clothes so with vinegar as to keep them always moist: and if the smell of any of those she waited upon was more than ordinary offensive, she snuffed vinegar up her nose and sprinkled vinegar upon her head clothes, and held a handkerchief wetted with vinegar up to her mouth.
(D. Defoe, *A Journal of the Plague Year*, Dent, 1966, pp. 88 and 101)

Although Defoe's is a fictional account of the plague, the remedies he mentions — especially the use of vinegar to 'clean' money and as an 'air freshener' — were authentic and employed well into the middle of the last century.

Questions and activities

1 Discuss those elements in reaction to the plague which would be considered rational and irrational according to contemporary standards.
2 The tabloid media have tended to use plague metaphors in their coverage of Aids. How valid is the comparison, and to what degree does Aids fit the moral panic paradigm?

Reading 3 An old wives' tale

On April Fool's Day, 1717, the wife of the British Ambassador at Constantinpole, Lady Mary Wortley Montague, wrote a letter to a friend at home in which she described how: the smallpox, so fatal and general amongst us, is here entirely harmless, by the invention of engrafting which is the term they give it. There is a set of old women, who make it their business to perform the operation, every autumn, in the month of September, when the great heat is abated. People send to one another to know if any of their family has a mind to have the smallpox; they make parties for this purpose, and when they are met (commonly fifteen or sixteen together) the old woman comes with a nut-shell of the matter of the best sort of smallpox, and asks what veins you please to have opened. She immediately rips open that you offer to her, with a large needle (which gives you no more pain than a common scratch) and puts into the vein as much matter as can lie upon the head of her needle. . . . Every year thousands undergo this operation, and the French Ambassador says pleasantly that they take the smallpox here by way of diversion, as they take the waters in other countries. There is no example of anyone that has died of it, and you may believe that I am well satisfied of the safety of this experiment since I intend to try it on my dear little son.

(Letter quoted in B. Inglis, *The History of Medicine*, Hodder & Stoughton, 1968, p. 111).

For centuries, a Chinese method for preventing smallpox had been to blow dried matter from smallpox scabs in powder form up the noses of healthy people. The efficacy of these practices would depend upon the state of the matter used, the risks of subsidiary infection and the accuracy of the initial diagnosis.

Questions and activities

1 Compile a list of Old Wives' and Old Doctors' Tales. (You might like to consider what advice they offer regarding women's complaints and childhood disorders.)
2 Make a list of alternative and complementary therapies, and explain the recent revival of interest in unorthodox healing.

Reading 4 Heroic medicine

[The last days of Charles II] Sixteen ounces of blood were removed from a vein in his right arm with immediate good effect. As was the approved practice at this time, the King was allowed to remain in the chair in which the convulsions seized him; his teeth were held forcibly open to prevent him biting his tongue; the regimen was, as Roger North pithily describes it, 'first to get him to wake, and then to keep him from sleeping' . . . cupping-glasses were applied to his shoulders and deep scarification carried out, by which they succeeded in removing another eight ounces of blood. A strong antimonial emetic was administered, but as the King could be got to swallow only a small portion of it, they determined to render assurance doubly sure by a full dose of Sulphate of Zinc. Strong purgatives were given, and supplemented by a succession of clysters. The hair was shorn close and pungent blistering agents applied all over his head; and as though this were not enough, the red-hot cautery was requisitioned as well. So severe were the convulsions that the physicians at first despaired of his life, but in some two hours consciousness was completely restored.

(B. Inglis, *The History of Medicine*, p. 102)

Historians tell us that King Charles II died from a heart attack.

Questions and activities

1 What was involved in the transition from heroic medicine to scientific medicine? Is it true to say that elements of heroic medicine persist in the attitude that the only effective treatment is a nasty one?
2 Discuss the social significance of the professionalisation of medicine.

Reading 5 Cancer

Writing about the significance of disease and illness as metaphors for social problems, Susan Sontag compares the meanings associated with tuberculosis in the nineteenth century with cancer today: two diseases 'spectacularly and similarly encumbered with metaphor'. She says that cancer provokes feelings of revulsion and helplessness in both the healthy and the ill. Cancer is associated with processes of decay and degradation and is subjected to rituals of denial, concealment and purification.

> When, not so many decades ago, learning that one had TB was tantamount to hearing a sentence of death — as today, in the popular imagination cancer equals death — it was common to conceal the identity of their disease from tuberculars and, after they had died, from their children. Even with patients informed about their disease, doctors and family were reluctant to talk freely. 'Verbally, I did not learn anything definite,' Kafka wrote to a friend in April 1924, from the sanatorium where he died two months later, 'since in discussing tuberculosis . . . everybody drops into a shy, evasive, glassy-eyed manner of speech.' Conventions of concealment with cancer are even more strenuous. . . . All this lying to and by cancer patients is a measure of how much harder it has become in advanced industrial societies

to come to terms with death. As death is now an offensively meaningless event, so that disease widely considered a synonym for death is experienced as something to hide. The policy of equivocating about the nature of their disease with cancer patients reflects the conviction that dying people are best spared the news that they are dying, and that the good death is the sudden one, best of all if it happens when we are unconscious or *asleep*.

(Susan Sontag, *Illness as Metaphor*, Penguin, 1978, pp. 11—12)

Questions and activities

1 How far do you agree with Sontag's view that cancer is seen as a verdict, a moral judgement of one's life?
2 Compile a list of the risk factors in cancer. Classify the factors into life-style and other factors.
3 Evaluate the effectiveness of the advertising compaigns against heroin and Aids, and devise some advertisements specifically aimed at young smokers and young drinkers.

Reading 6 Living standards and the working class in nineteenth-century England

As with clothing, so with food. The workers get what is too bad for the property-holding class. In the great towns of England everything may be had of the best, but it costs money; and the workman, who must keep house on a couple of pence, cannot afford much expense. Moreover, he usually receives his wages on a Saturday evening, for, although a beginning has been made in the payment of wages on Friday, this excellent arrangement is by no means universal; and so he comes to market at five or even seven o'clock, while the buyers of the middle-class have had the first choice during the morning, when the market teems with the best of everything. But when the workers reach it the best has vanished, and, if it was still there, they would probably not be able to buy it. The potatoes which the workers buy are usually poor, the vegetables wilted, the cheese old and of poor quality, the bacon rancid, the meat lean, tough, taken from old, often diseased cattle, or such as have died a natural death, and not fresh even then, often half-decayed. The sellers are usually small hucksters who buy up inferior goods, and can sell them cheaply for reason of their badness. The poorest workers are forced to use still another device to get together the things they need with their few pence. As nothing can be sold on a Sunday, and all shops must be closed at twelve o'clock on Saturday night, such things as would not keep until Monday are sold at any price between ten o'clock and midnight. But nine-tenths of what is sold at ten o'clock is past using by Sunday morning, yet these are precisely the provisions which make up the Sunday dinner of the poorest class. . . .

But they are victimised in another way by the money-greed of the middle-class. Dealers and manufacturers adulterate all kinds of provisions in an atrocious manner, and without the slightest regard to the health of consumers. We have heard 'The Manchester Guardian' upon this subject, let us hear another organ of the middle-class – 'The Liverpool Mercury': 'Salted butter is sold for fresh, the lumps being covered with a coating of fresh butter, or a pound of fresh being laid on top to taste, while the salted article is sold after this test, or the whole mass is washed and then sold as fresh. With sugar, pounded rice and other cheap adulterating materials are mixed, and the whole is sold at full price. The refuse of soap-boiling establishments is also mixed with other things and sold as sugar. Chicory and other cheap stuff is mixed with ground coffee, and artificial coffee beans with the unground article. Cocoa is often adulterated with fine brown earth, treated with fat to render it more easily mistakable for real cocoa. Tea is mixed with the leaves of the sloe and with other refuse, or dried tea-leaves are roasted on hot copper plates, so returning to the proper colour and being sold as fresh. Pepper is mixed with pounded nutshells; port-wine is manufactured outright (out of alcohol and dyestuffs) and it is notorious that more of it is consumed in England alone than is produced in Portugal; and tobacco is mixed with disgusting substances of all sorts and in all possible forms in which the article is produced.

(F. Engels, *The Condition of the Working Class in England*, Lawrence & Wishart, 1954, p. 102–4)

Questions and activities

1 Engels is here attempting to show how life-style and choice are structured by socio-economic factors. What would this

approach tell us about the diet of the poor and the old today?
2 Complete your own diet sheet for a week, listing mealtimes and the quantities and types of foods eaten. What are the characteristics of the children's food market? How are our food preferences shaped?

Reading 7   Smoking

In her book *The Ladykillers* Bobbie Jacobson writes that although the proportion of men who smoke is going down, the proportion of women smokers has remained stable because any reduction in numbers through women giving up cigarettes is cancelled out by young women starting. Further, women smokers smoke more cigarettes than men. Men have tended to respond to the reports on smoking and health by either stopping altogether or cutting their consumption. She says that different factors are involved in each stage of a 'smoking career'; the factors persuading people to start smoking are different from those which encourage people to persist or to cease. Different factors apply in the case of men and women. Women, for example, have a greater emotional investment in smoking than men because it helps them to contain feelings of frustration and anger which women are inhibited from expressing because such feelings are considered unladylike and because women's opportunities to tackle the sources of their anger are structurally limited. Women who try to give up smoking get less support within the family than do men. Women expect, and are expected, to 'cope'. Further, for many women giving up is made more difficult because of the fear of getting fat and because of the positive images of women-smokers presented by the advertising media:

> Every woman who discussed her smoking problem with me was convinced she was 'hooked' on nicotine. By far the most important criteria for establishing whether a drug is physically addictive are the phenomena of 'tolerance' and 'withdrawal syndrome' which are characteristic of narcotic drugs such as barbiturates and opiates (morphine-like drugs). 'Tolerance' means that as drug-use continues, the drug-taker becomes 'dependent' and needs more of the drug to achieve the desired effect. The 'withdrawal syndrome', by contrast, results from

sudden stoppage of the drug supply; the nerves affected by the drug become overactive during a possibly unpleasant but short re-adaptation period. Nicotine fits some, but not all the criteria for physical dependence. Smokers who experiment with the occasional cigarette rapidly begin to tolerate the nausea and headiness that smoking causes. They soon find themselves smoking more and more — needing to smoke every day (only 2 per cent of all smokers remain truly occasional smokers). Yet they don't keep on stepping up the 'dose' of nicotine and usually settle for between 10 and 25 cigarettes a day. Indeed the amount smoked seems so much a reflection of economic and social pressures as internal chemical forces. When people try to stop smoking they may well experience unpleasant 'withdrawal symptoms' but unlike narcotic addicts who stop, many don't . . . the difficulty many smokers experience in stopping could also be psychological or social in origin. Indeed when the motivation to stop is very high, such as an increase in tax on cigarettes or in smokers who have a heart attack, the success rate for stopping can more than double. Perhaps the strongest challenge to the idea of straightforward nicotine addiction is the simple observation that social status is a more important determinant of who smokes and who stops than either psychological or physiological makeup. To invoke nicotine dependence to explain why doctors have found it easier to give up smoking than labourers, and indeed why women find it harder to give up smoking than men, you would have to support the unlikely proposition that there is something about being a doctor (or a man) that confers physiological resistance to the addictive pull of tobacco.

(*The Ladykillers*, Pluto, 1981, pp. 24–26)

Questions and activities

1 Why is smoking a feminist issue?
2 What questions does this passage raise about the concept of addiction?

Read the following two passages and then consider:

1 the pattern and causes of ill health in poor countries, and
2 the barriers to the WHO target of 'Health for all by the year 2000'

Reading 8 Infant feeding

War on Want's research demonstrating the impact of Western baby-food promotion on the health of children in poor countries resulted in the introduction of a code of marketing in 1979. It had found that advertisements for dried cow's milk claimed it was superior to human milk and that artificial baby foods were being officially and commercially promoted in the forms of free clinic equipment, commercially sponsored 'nursery assistants', free samples of baby foods and glossy advertisements aimed at mothers anxious to give their children a good start in life in countries where many fail to reach their first birthday.

All over the world, women living in areas without a pure supply of water and the means to sterilise bottles and teats had been switching to bottle-feeding. Babies were suffering and dying from gastric disorders because their milk was contaminated by infected water. Milk was being improperly mixed because mothers were unable to read or understand the instructions on the tins and also lacked the appropriate measuring spoons. Processed milk is expensive relative to family incomes (baby-milk is 2 per cent of the British average wage, it can be anything from 10 per cent–80 per cent in some poor countries) and many mothers economised by mixing weak feeds. Too concentrated, the feed will raise sodium levels to a dangerous point, too weak and the baby is starving.

Importing canned cow's milk to feed babies drains a country's reserves and the cost of self-sufficiency in dried milk demands livestock, processing and packaging plant – India, for example would require a herd of 114 million extra cows. In some poor countries doctors and governments are now actively promoting natural feeding. In Chile for example, the campaign to persuade mothers to feed babies with human rather than cow milk is credited with the fall in infant mortality from 180/1000 to 47/1000 between 1967 and 1977. In 1972 6 per cent of infants were breastfed after 6 months, in 1977 18 per cent were.

(U. Dobraszczyc, unpublished paper)

Reading 9 Infant health care

Describing the return of a child, Batista João, to his village in Mozambique after treatment for cholera, Muller says that his care illustrates the concept of primary health care as it has been conceived in that country:

1 it reaches past the towns into the rural areas;
2 it focuses on prevention of disease in the community, not on an individual cure;
3 it depends upon a team approach by sufficiently trained, organised and motivated health workers and not upon highly trained and specialised doctors;
4 it has access to specialised services and equipment where necessary;
5 health care is not the responsibility of one group of workers: it involves political organisations, state farms, private traders and even the local water company.

No doctors were involved. Batista João's diagnosis [of cholera] and treatment had been carried out entirely by health workers whose maximum formal qualification was six years' schooling followed by a two-year course for 'agentes de medicina' or 'agentes de medicina preventiva'. Both the treatment and preventative health work were carried out according to the guidelines established at national level with resources and guidance from the provincial health directorate. The only intervention by a doctor was the initiative of the medical director from the neighbouring district in calling me to look at the water supply; to diagnose and treat not an individual symptom but a collective hazard affecting the whole community. In many districts of Mozambique, this responsibility is executed by 'tecnicos de medicina' — they have nine years' schooling and three year's general medical training.

This study puts flesh on the bones of a concept that is much talked about but sometimes little understood, that of 'primary health care'. China's 'barefoot doctors' are the best-known example, but too often they are described in terms of the health care they provide, without sufficient reference to the organisational structures and philosophies on which they are based.

(M. Muller, *The Health of Nations*, Pluto, 1983, p. 126)

Reading 10 Class and the NHS

Below are two accounts of the relationships between class and the NHS. Iliffe presents the establishment of the NHS as a class —

gender victory, whereas Walters sees it as the outcome of a broad political consensus and a means to defuse class conflict.

1 From the formation of the Ministry of Health in 1919, to the creation of the NHS in 1948, women and labour formed a coalition of interests aiming to expand and organise a jumble of medical services run by central and local government, by charitable organisations, by insurance committees, and through the Poor Law. At the end of the First World War a working-class family could receive medical care from as many as nine different doctors working under five different organisations. The working man would see his panel doctor for all illnesses apart from tuberculosis. His wife, if she was insured, would see the same panel doctor for all illnesses apart from TB (from which 40 000 people died a year) and problems in childbirth. If she was not insured then she could see a private doctor, if she could afford it, or, if she was too poor, a parish doctor (provided under Poor Law Regulations) or a doctor from a medical charity. During pregnancy she would use the municipal maternity service, and at her confinement would be attended by a midwife or a doctor from this service. Any member of the family who contracted TB would receive treatment from a local government TB officer. Infants and children under school age would be looked after by the maternity centre doctor. After they had gone to school they would be attended for 'school diseases' by the school medical officer, and by a private doctor (who was also the family's panel doctor) when they were too ill to go to school. After school age and up to sixteen they would use the private doctor, but after sixteen they would be able to see the same doctor under the panel system.

(S. Iliffe, *The NHS — a Picture of Health?* Lawrence & Wishart, 1983, pp. 20−21)

Walters argues that the NHS originated in several forces but that:

2 there is little evidence that working class patients were singularly disadvantaged in their access to medical care before 1948 and working class pressures for reform were neither strong nor did they envisage comprehensive changes in the organisation and delivery of health care.

She argues that class politics were less important in framing the

NHS than the need for the state and the professions to respond to the fiscal and organisational problems of the pre-war health services. War brought the problems to a head and showed a way out through the centralised system of the emergency medical services. The chief victims of the pre-war system had been the middle-class. The key element in Walters' account of the NHS is not working-class struggle but middle-class power and need. But, like Iliffe, she argues that the state acted, not as an 'honest broker' but as a participant in class conflict defused by the NHS.

Moreover because the NHS removed the direct cost of health care, and in theory, provided care to all people irrespective of their means, it gave rise to the notion that class inequalities in health would diminish. In these ways the state has served an ideological function, in that it has helped to create a belief in the decline of class inequalities and permitted an interpretation of continuing inequalities in terms which emphasise the individual's responsibility for his or her own health.

(V. Walters, *Class Inequality and Health Care*, Croom Helm, 1980, pp. 156 and 160)

Questions and activities

1 Compile accounts of health care and illness from older people whose memories go back to the period before the establishment of the NHS.
2 Evaluate the concept of class struggle in relation to the NHS today.
3 In what respects can the NHS be seen as the embodiment of the 'welfare principle'?

Readings 11 and 12 both present critiques of medical care. Illich's is a cultural critique because he argues against medicine in its contemporary form, and Tudor Hart's is materialist because he does not challenge medicine as such, rather its pattern of distribution.

Reading 11   Iatrogenesis

The undesirable side-effects of approved, mistaken, callous, or contraindicated technical contacts with the medical system represent just the first level of pathogenic medicine. Such clinical iatrogenesis includes not only the damage that doctors inflict with the intention of curing or of exploiting the patient, but also those other torts [wrongs] that result from the doctor's attempt to protect himself against the possibility of a suit for malpractice. Such attempts to avoid litigation and prosecution may now do more damage than any other iatrogenic stimulus.

On a second level, medical practice sponsors sickness by reinforcing a morbid society that encourages people to become consumers of curative, preventive, industrial and environmental medicine. Second-level iatrogenesis finds its expression in various symptoms of social overmedicalisation . . . social iatrogenesis. . . .

On a third level, the so-called health professions have an even deeper, culturally health-denying effect in so far as they destroy the potential of people to deal with their human weakness, vulnerability, and uniqueness in a personal and autonomous way.

(I. Illich, *Medical Nemesis*, Bantam Books, 1977, pp. 32–4)

Reading 12 The Inverse Care Law

In areas with most sickness and death, general practitioners have more work, larger lists, less hospital support, and inherit more clinically ineffective traditions of consultation, than in the healthiest areas; and hospital doctors shoulder heavier case-loads with less staff and equipment, more obsolete buildings, and suffer recurrent crises in the availability of beds and replacement staff. These trends can be summed up as the Inverse Care Law: that the availability of good medical care tends to vary inversely with the need of the population served.

If the NHS had continued to adhere to its original principles, with construction of health centres a first priority in industrial areas, all financed from taxation rather than direct flat-rate contribution, free at the time of use, and fully inclusive of all personal health services, including family-planning, the operation of the Inverse Care Law would have been modified much more than it has been; but even the service as it is has been effective in redistributing care, considering the powerful social forces operating against this. If our health service had evolved as a free-market, or even on a fee-for-item-of-service basis pre-paid by private insurance, the law would have operated much more completely than it does; our situation might approximate to that in the United States, with the added disadvantage of smaller national wealth. The force that creates and maintains the Inverse Care Law is the operation of the market, and its cultural and ideological superstructure that has permeated the thought and directed the ambitions of the profession during all of its modern history. The more health services are removed from the force of the market, the more successful we can be in redistributing care away from its 'natural' distribution in a market economy; but this will be a redistribution, an intervention to correct a fault natural to our form of society, and therefore incompletely successful and politically unstable, in the absence of more fundamental social change.

(Dr J. Tudor Hart, *The Lancet*, 27 February 1971)

Questions and activities

1 Outline and evaluate Illich's concept of iatrogenesis.
2 In what respects is it true to say that those with the greatest need get the least medical care?

Reading 13 Colds and chills – some old wives' tales

C. Helman, an anthropologist and a GP, was interested in the origin of the saying 'Starve a fever and feed a cold', so he examined the folk beliefs of some Londoners about colds and chills.

Wind at body temperature is not dangerous, and is merely 'fresh air'. Night air is however considered dangerous, especially by older patients. Some areas of skin are seen as more vulnerable than others to penetration by environmental cold – particularly the top of the head, the back of the neck and the feet. 'Colds' occurred when these areas were inadvertently exposed to draughts or damp: 'getting your feet wet'; 'walking round with damp hair'; 'going out into the rain without a hat on'. (Temperature changes between hot and cold environments as well as sudden seasonal temperature changes – coming back to Britain from a Spanish holiday – cause 'colds'.) 'Cold', once it has entered the body can move around. From damp feet it can migrate and cause a 'stomach chill' or it can shift even further upwards to cause a 'head cold' or a 'sinus cold'. In general 'chills' occur below the waist ('stomach chill', 'bladder chill', 'kidney chill') and 'colds' above it ('a head cold', or 'a cold in the sinuses', 'a cold in the chest').

Unlike 'fevers', 'colds' and 'chills' are more one's own responsibility. They are the result of carelessness or lack of foresight — if 'you don't dress properly', 'you allow your head to get wet', 'wash your hair when you don't feel well'.

(C. Helman 'Feed a Cold, Starve a Fever — Folk Models of Infection in an English Suburban Community and Their Relation to Medical treatment', *Culture Medicine and Psychiatry*, 2, 1978, pp. 111–13)

Questions and activities

1 Examine the role of euphemism in clinical consultations and the scientific and lay dimensions of conditions such as 'trouble with my nerves' and 'having a weak stomach'.

There is truth in the assertion that 'the separate worlds of experience and reference of the layman and the professional worker are always in potential conflict with one another' (Freidson). However, it is important not to overemphasise the distinctions between lay, folk and professional systems of medical thought since they may coexist and even overlap. One of the barriers to effective clinical practice may be the assumption that patients are either ignorant or unable to understand the professional approach despite the fact that we are all subject to a process of socialisation around the bio-medical model. In any case, medical theory and clinical practice are separate realms, and there are occasions when professionals readily adopt lay and folk approaches to medical problems.

2 Compare the sociological approach to illness with the bio-medical approach.
3 What is meant by (w)holistic medicine?

Reading 14   Doctor-patient interaction

One of the 2500 GPs whose consultations were taped, with permission, by P. Byrne and B. Long described the pressures on doctors in the following way:

> The doctor's primary task is to manage his time. If he allows patients to rabbit on about their conditions then the doctor will

lose control of time and will spend all his time sitting in the surgery listening to irrelevant rubbish. Effective doctoring is characterised by a quick, clean job. (In a morning surgery this doctor will see patients at a rate of one every five minutes. His appointment system schedules up to 14 per hour and, he claims, people rarely have to wait long.)

(P. Byrne and B. Long, *Doctors Talking to Patients*, DHSS, 1976, p. 93)

Three-quarters of the consultations were doctor-centred, in that the practitioner ignored verbal leads from the patient and concentrated on eliciting answers to his own closed questions. The researchers present the doctor-centred and patient-centred consultation as examples of personal style which did not vary with the social characteristics of patients. However, other researchers have found class- and gender-related differences.

Questions and activities

1 To what degree do doctor-centred and patient-centred styles of interaction represent different models of the therapeutic relationship?
2 Discuss the interaction routines commonly used by participants in medical settings.

Reading 15 Health and gender roles

In a test of the arguments that clinical judgements about the traits characterising healthy individuals vary according to the sex of the person being judged and that clinical judgments parallel sex-role stereotypes, Broverman and Broverman concluded:

On the face of it, the finding that clinicians tend to ascribe more male-valued stereotypic traits to healthy men than to healthy women may seem trite. However, an examination of the content of these items suggests that this trite-seeming phenomenon conceals a powerful, negative assessment of women. For instance, among these items, clinicians are more likely to suggest that healthy women differ from healthy men by being more submissive; less independent; less adventurous; more easily influenced; less aggressive; less competitive; more excitable in minor crises; having their feelings more easily hurt; being more emotional; more conceited about their appearance; less objective and disliking maths and science. This constellation seems a most unusual way of describing a mature healthy individual.

(I. K. Broverman and D. M. Broverman *et al.*, 'Sex-role Stereotypes and Clinical Judgements of Mental Health', *Journal of Consulting and Clinical Psychiatry*, vol. 34, 1970, pp. 1–7)

Questions and activities

1 A test of sex stereotyping can be made by subdividing a group of people into two halves and presenting each half with a list of attributes − such as independence, intelligence, talkativeness, vanity, reliability, caring, insecurity, consideration and so on. One half is asked to consider the positive and negative dimensions of these attributes and then to rank them, and the other half of the group is asked to indicate which are normally associated with each gender. Compare the decisions of the sub-groups in relation to each other and in relation to the gender of members.
2 Examine the relationships between stereotypings and the health care of (a) women and (b) members of ethnic minorities.

Reading 16 Illness as deviance

If illness is to be shown to violate some normative rule, it must be shown that society does not expect its members either to fall ill, where this means to have illness conditions, or to occupy the status sick and thus perform the sick role. We certainly do not expect people to refrain from illness condition in the same way as we expect them not to commit a crime or be sinful. No person, however hard he tries, can guarantee to avoid illness. Nor do we even expect those who are in the business of controlling illness to go through life without having any illness. While we may expect a judge not to commit a crime or a vicar not to commit one of the seven deadly sins, we cannot expect a doctor or health educator not to be ill.

(D. Robinson, *The Process of Becoming Ill*, RKP, 1971, p. 93)

Questions and activities

1 Outline the concept of the **sick role**.

2 Assess Parsons' view (pages 65–7) that sickness is a form of deviancy in the light of Robinson's observations.
3 Compare the social identities associated with minor illness, serious illness, handicap, chronic illness and terminal illness.

Reading 17 Kinship and friendship

Many researchers have found it useful to distinguish between lay referral, intervention and consultation in order to examine the forms of assistance and the personnel actually involved in the non-professional treatment of illness. Some writers argue that kin and friendship groups perform different functions in this regard. For example, a summary of the findings on the influence of kinship and friendship networks on the use of maternity services by eighty-eight working-class Scottish women:

> Differences emerged between the utilizers and the underutilizers regarding aspects of the kin and friendship sectors of their social networks and from questions concerning lay referral and lay consultation for various hypothetical but commonly occurring problem situations. It appears that utilizers made greater use of friends and husbands and less use of mothers and or other relatives, and tended to consult a narrower range of lay consultants. These findings were consistent with, and perhaps reinforced, observed differences in their network structure. Underutilizers appeared to rely more on a variety of readily available relatives and friends as lay consultants. There appeared to be only one large interlocking network within which the underutilizers obtained the majority of their advice. Utilizers, on the other hand, had separate or differentiated kin and friendship networks . . . and appeared to be relatively independent of both.
> (J. McKinlay, 'Social Networks, lay consultations and help-seeking behaviour', *Social Forces*, 1973, 5, pp. 275–92)

Questions

1 What is involved in going to the doctor?
2 Compare lay and professional methods of consultation, diagnosis and treatment in matters of sickness and health.

Reading 18 People in hospital

Surveys of patients have found, in the case of hospital patients, that 64 per cent were very satisfied with their medical care and 69 per cent with the nursing staff (Gallup, 1984), and in the case of surgery visits 90 per cent of patients were satisfied with the care they received (A. Cartwright and R. Anderson, *General Practice Re-visited*, Tavistock, 1981). Nevertheless there are significant areas of complaint from both groups of patients. The Royal Commission on the NHS 1978 found the following sources of dissatisfaction among hospital patients.

Reason	% dissatisfied
Information about progress	25
Length of time in hospital	19
Length of wait before seeing a doctor	16
Difficulty in understanding the doctor	15

The patients found the following deficiencies in general practice:

Reason	% dissatisfied
Comfort of the waiting room	30
Adequacy of explanations	23
Keeping people waiting	21
Taking time and not hurrying the patient	14
Examining the patient carefully	13

Questions and activities

1 How appropriate is Goffman's concept of the total institution to hospitals?
2 In what ways might the demands of medical bureaucracies interfere with medical care?

Reading 19 Medical models of pregnancy and childbirth

Medical models of pregnancy have changed over the last 150 years. Despite high maternal and infant mortality rates, childbirth was traditionally viewed as a natural process involving other people only at the time of delivery. A combination of superstition, prudery, ignorance and theories about the proper roles of men and women, meant that it was an exclusively female concern. Today, childbirth is medically monitored from the point of conception by a predominantly male profession. Childbirth has been medicalised, institutionalised and industrialised (through the development of artificial reproduction techniques) and the mortality rates associated with it have declined. These two classes of development are not causally connected and the strongest causal factors are improved diets and living standards.

The medical frame of reference
In talking about the different ways in which doctors and mothers view pregnancy, we are talking about a fundamental difference in their perspectives on the meaning of childbearing. It is not simply a difference of opinion about approach and procedures – about whether pregnancy is normal or pathological, or whether or not labours should be routinely induced. Rather we are suggesting that doctors and mothers have a qualitatively different way of looking at the nature, context and management of reproduction. We use the concept of a *frame of reference* to indicate this difference. 'Frame of reference' embraces both the notion of an ideological perspective – a system of values and attitudes through which mothers and doctors view pregnancy – and of a reference group – a network of individuals who are significant influences upon these sets of attitudes and values.
(A. Oakley and H. Graham in H. Roberts (ed.), *Women, Health and Reproduction*, RKP, 1981, p. 50)

Five major features of the MFR are identified:

1 Reproduction is viewed as a medical specialism with expertise held by doctors whose approach marks an advance from the superstition and ignorance of previous years.
2 Pregnancy has a paradoxical character in as much as it is a natural function which can be accomplished successfully only in a controlled environment away from the rest of the woman's social world. All pregnancies are treated as though they were going to be abnormal unless proved otherwise. The 'treatment rule' of general medicine means that procedures introduced to deal with abnormal pregnancy will become routine.
3 The success of the event is judged by technical criteria such as neo-natal mortality and maternal death rates. Qualitative

criteria may be paramount for the mother and those professionals concerned with post-natal care and maternal bonding but they are not uppermost in the delivery room.
4 Reproduction is divorced from its social context and pregnancy is the only salient status for the woman patient. Her other obligations and roles are not only irrelevant but a threat to medical authority.
5 Women's identities are determined primarily by their domestic roles. To succumb to biology and have babies is not only natural but the chief source of a woman's fulfilment. The reality is that women are unprepared for the responsibility and isolation that motherhood brings. The medical frame of reference casts women in a passive and subordinate role and focuses upon the event of birth, leaving women unsupported and unprepared in motherhood itself.

Questions and activities

1 Discuss the changes that have occurred in women's experiences of childbirth and motherhood over the last fifty years.
2 Review the advice literature on maternity which is published for the non-medical reader.
3 What support does Reading 20 give for the notion that medicine is mysogynist?

Reading 20 Social invalidation

Any situation involving the assumption or attribution of mental illness is an exercise in social invalidation . . . Invalidation is done in two ways, by labelling and by physical restraint. Labelling includes diagnosis as well as the application of words meaning ill, foreign, strange or no good by one person against another. Physical restraint includes external coercion such as strait-jackets and hospitalization and internal control by means of drugs, electricity or surgery.

Labelling is most effective when performed by professionals in socially accepted and expected settings — the doctor's office, the hospital emergency room or the courtroom. However, labelling is influential in other circumstances because it essentially consists of the magical use of words to control an anxiety-provoking person. Such a person is one who breaks social rules, primarily prevailing standards of moral and social intercourse.

This leads the rule breaker to become the recipient of others' projections and the focus of their disassociated perversity and self-hatred.

Labelling is an interpersonal manoeuvre which enables a number of people, ranging from a family and its agents to a society and its agencies, to deny what they feel and to attack anyone who would arouse these denied *feelings*.

(J. H. Berke, *I Haven't Had to Go Mad Here*, Penguin, 1979, pp. 19–24 *passim*)

Questions and activities

1 To what extent does Berke, in this piece, broaden the concept of labelling and give it a psychological dimension which is not found in the work of other writers?
2 Examine Scheff's contention that concepts of madness are acquired in childhood, and review the images of abnormality, craziness and so on presented in children's television programmes.
3 What can sociological approaches contribute to our understanding of mental illness?

Reading 21 Women and health care

Although the sociology of nursing is still an undeveloped area, three observations can be drawn from the work of Celia Davies and Eva Gamarnikow:

1 Nursing developed as a respectable occupation for women from good background on the analogy of the Victorian bourgeois family – the doctor being the equivalent of the paterfamilias and the qualified nurse the mother with her own separate sphere of authority over the ward staff (maids) and the patients (children) subject ultimately to his.
2 The status of nursing relative to doctoring was initially given a boost by the acceptance of the germ theory of disease reflected in the Nightingale stress on hygiene, nursing the ward and letting nature take its course under the watchful eye of the trained nurse. However, despite technical and scientific changes in nursing practice, improvements in its socio-economic status have been retarded by the continued stress on the hygiene

element and the Nightingale concept of vocation – 'You don't go into nursing for the money'.
3 The qualities associated with good nursing are the opposite of those associated with good doctoring.

The significance of gender in health care is illustrated by the findings of the inquiry by the Women's National Commission, *Women and the Health Service* (Cabinet Office, 1986), some of which are given below:

82.5 per cent of the sample of almost 6 000 women would use a Well Woman Clinic if there was one in their area.
72 per cent wanted to be able to choose whether they were treated by a male of female doctor for hospital treatment, but only 18 per cent thought it mattered in general practice.

Preference for advice

	male doctor	female doctor	no pref	nurse
gynaecological	5.3	42.0	51.0	0.9
family planning	4.2	36.3	55.7	3.8
maternity care	5.6	25.2	61.0	8.2
other health problems	10.7	9.1	79.9	0.5
care of children	8.4	6.6	83.4	1.6
care of elderly relative	9.1	7.4	80.2	3.3

Of those who would prefer to see a female doctor for *any* aspect of health care (46 per cent), the rank order of reasons was (1) better understanding of your problems (37 per cent), (2) find it easier and less embarrassing to talk to her (31 per cent), (3) she would be more sympathetic and caring (14 per cent).
Eighty-five per cent of women would like more information about how to keep themselves and their families healthy. The rank ordering of their concerns were (1) mental health, including stress and depression (48 per cent); (2) diet (46 per cent); and (3) vaccinations and preventative health care (45 per cent).

Question

1 How does gender affect caring roles?

Glossary of specialist terms

aetiology: both the study of the causation of illness and of the aggregate of factors that contribute to it.

chemical therapeutics: drug-based treatments for disease. In 1909 Paul Ehrlich coined the term 'magic bullet' when looking forward to drugs to be directed at a single target of infection or site of infection. In the event, the development of antibiotics has resulted in preparations which act against a broad rather than a narrow spectrum.

high-yield strains: new, heavy-cropping cereals and grains with yields 4 or 5 times these of the indigenous cereals they replaced. Their disadvantages are that they demand higher levels of fertiliser, irrigation and chemical protection than native seeds, so their related costs are high.

green revolution: name given to the programme of selective plant breeding started in the 1940s. It resulted in high-yield strains or varieties (HYV) of seeds and was expected to eradicate world hunger. On reflection, it appears that the benefits of HYVs depend on a technological approach to farming which has increased the hold of international food firms (agribusiness) over food production in Third World countries.

pharmacopoeia: stock of drugs and also the published list of available drugs and advice on treatment. In 1933 the British Pharmacopoeia contained only 36 synthetic drugs.

placebo: literally meaning 'I shall be pleasing', it refers to preparations which please rather than medicinally benefit the patient. In the early 1930s there was a 3-year randomised control trial in which a group of angina patients tried out 13 new drugs while a control group were given bicarbonate of soda. By all measures of effectiveness the bicarb was most successful – suggesting that what the patient believes about treatment may be more important than the treatment itself.

polypharmacy: tendency to prescribe a collection of drugs from the vast range available.

sulpha drugs, sulphonamides: before the development of antibiotics, the main hope against infection was immunisation, which stimulated the body's immune system. In 1932 a preparation was developed from a dyestuff which was seen to have anti-bacterial properties – Prontosil. Unlike antiseptics which destroyed body tissue along with bacteria, the sulpha drugs simply acted upon bacteria. Their success generated considerable commercial interest in drug research, prompted medical people to reconsider chemotherapy, and stimulated the work which resulted in the development of the antibiotics.

Bibliography

A good general reader is still **D. Tuckett**, *An Introduction to Medical Sociology*, Tavistock, London, 1976.

L. Doyal and I. Pennell, *A Political Economy of Health*, Pluto Press, London, 1979, is a text which contains a good deal of comparative and historical material.

H. Graham, *Women, Health and the Family*, Wheatsheaf Books, London, 1984, is broad in its scope and empirical range and an excellent overview of health and related issues in the primary setting.

Other readings:

P. Chesler, *Women and Madness*, Allen Lane, London, 1974. An influential text.

A. Davis (ed.). *Relationships between Doctors and Patients*, Saxon House, Teakfield, London, 1978; and

D. Robinson, *Patients, Practitioners and Medical Care: Aspects of Medical Sociology*, Heinemann Medical Books, London, 1973; both give good accounts of doctor–patient interaction and the distinctive contribution that sociological approaches can make to sickness and health.

Texts that have begun to examine gender relationships in caring and healing are

C. Davies (ed.), *Re-writing Nursing History*, Croom Helm, London, 1980;

M. Stacey (ed.), *Health and the Division of Labour*, BSA, London, 1977; and

R. White, *Social Change and the Development of the Nursing Profession – a study of the Poor Law Nursing Service 1848–1948*, Henry Kimpton. London 1978;

E. Gamarnikow, 'Sexual Division of Labour – the Case of Nursing', in A. Kuhn and A. Wolpe, *Feminism and Materialism*, RKP, London, 1978, provides a very interesting account of the Nightingale reforms and the ideological climate in which they were accomplished.

I. Kennedy, *The Unmasking of Medicine*, Allen & Unwin, London, 1980, is the text of the Reith Lectures delivered by the author, a member of the legal profession, who airs a number of uncomfortable questions about the role of medicine in society.

N. Parry and J. Parry, *The Rise of the Medical Profession*, Croom Helm, London, 1970, is a sociological history of the development of institutionalised medicine in Britain.

P. Sedgwick, *Psycho Politics*, Pluto Press, London, 1982, reviews in depth sociological accounts of madness.

A. Clare, *Psychiatry in Dissent*, Tavistock, London, 1976 discusses sociological approaches alongside conventional medical and psychiatric accounts.

Index

affluence, diseases of 4
ageing 43–5
anaesthesia 13–14
asbestos 55–6

Bevan, A. 37
bio-medical model 57–8
Black Report 47–51
Brenner, H. 51
Brown, G. and Harris, T. 85

cancer 25, 53–5, 70, 106
cholera 10, 17, 22
cinderella populations 45
cinderella services 43–5
class, and access to health care 48
  and illness 48–51
  struggle and medicine 38–40, 112–14

death certificates 23–4
demography 26
deviance 65, 119, 123
diet 26–33, 107
doctors, interaction with patients 66–71, 81, 114, 117

epidemiology 13, 22–6
ethnicity 80–2

gender health and illness 82–5, 124
germ theory 11–13
Goffman, E. 77

health, and the role of medicine 8
homoeopathy 20
hospitals 16–17 (*see* National Health Service, total institution)

iatrogenesis, I.Illich 114–15
inverse care law 115–16

Kuhn, T. 9

Laing, R. D. 78–9

magic and witchcraft 102
maternity 14, 121–3 (*see* medicalisation of society)
medicalisation of society 72
medicine, and autonomy 40
  and the class structure 38, 112
  and power 72, 85
  as a profession 14, 19–20
  and social control 103
  and science 11–14
mental illness 73–85

National Health Service (NHS) 37–47

Parsons, T., and the sick role 65–7
personality and illness 53
prescriptions 4–6, 60–2
public health movement 26–31

referral 64–7 (*see also* trivial consultations, symptom iceberg)

Scheff, T. 76
sick role 51–2, 65
smoking 53–5, 109–10
sociology of illness 57–9
symptom iceberg 5, 62–4
Szasz, T. 75

Third World 33–6, 111–12
total institution 68–9, 77–8
tranquillisers 60–2
trivial consultations 59
Tudor Hart, J. 115
typifications, doctors of patients 62, 71
  patients of doctors 63, 68

unemployment and health 51–2, 86

World Health Organisation 26, 33–6